KEEP YOUR
BRAIN
STRONGER
FOR
LONGER

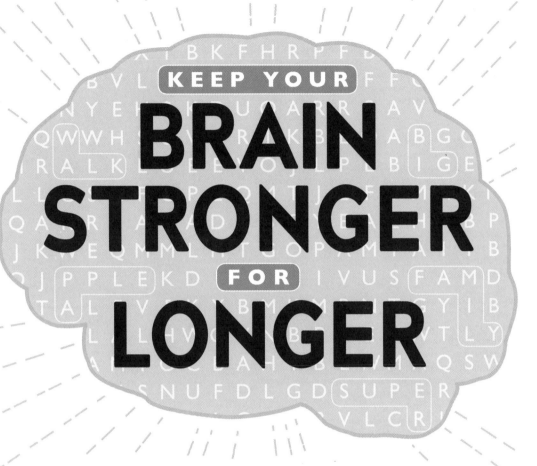

KEEP YOUR BRAIN STRONGER for LONGER

201 BRAIN-TEASING EXERCISES
for Anyone with Mild Cognitive Impairment

Tonia Vojtkofsky, PsyD

FOREWORD BY ROBERT G. FELDMAN, MD

THE EXPERIMENT

NEW YORK

KEEP YOUR BRAIN STRONGER FOR LONGER: *201 Brain-Teasing Exercises for Anyone with Mild Cognitive Impairment*
Copyright © 2015 Tonia Vojtkofsky
Foreword copyright © 2015 Robert G. Feldman

The Experiment, LLC
220 East 23rd Street, Suite 600
New York, NY 10010-4658
theexperimentpublishing.com

This book contains the opinions and ideas of its author. It is intended to provide helpful and informative material on the subjects addressed in the book. It is sold with the understanding that the author and publisher are not engaged in rendering medical, health, or any other kind of personal professional services in the book. The author and publisher specifically disclaim all responsibility for any liability, loss, or risk—personal or otherwise—that is incurred as a consequence, directly or indirectly, of the use and application of any of the contents of this book.

The Experiment's books are available at special discounts when purchased in bulk for premiums and sales promotions as well as for fund-raising or educational use. For details, contact us at info@theexperimentpublishing.com.

Library of Congress Cataloging-in-Publication Data:
Vojtkofsky, Tonia.
  Keep your brain stronger for longer : 201 brain exercises for people with mild cognitive impairment / Tonia Vojtkofsky, Psy.D. ; foreword by Robert G. Feldman, MD.
     pages cm
  ISBN 978-1-61519-262-5 (pbk.)
  1. Mind and body. 2. Brain. 3. Mild cognitive impairment. I. Title.
  BF151.V65 2015
  158.1--dc23
                                    2014037099

ISBN 978-1-61519-262-5

Cover design by Beth Bugler
Text design by Pauline Neuwirth, Neuwirth & Associates, Inc.

Manufactured in the United States of America

First printing July 2015
10 9 8 7 6 5 4 3

KEEP YOUR
BRAIN
STRONGER
FOR
LONGER

CONTENTS

FOREWORD

by Robert G. Feldman, MD

I FIRST MET TONIA VOJTKOFSKY when she came to my office to tell me about her new company, Cognitive Care Solutions, and its innovative treatment plan. As a primary care physician, and consultant for patients with dementia for the past twenty-five years, I have seen many fads come and go. Dr. Vojtkofsky began by pulling out a sheet titled *Cognitive Enhancement Therapy—Targeting Modifiable Risk Factors for Brain Health*, which listed lifestyle features such as nutrition, physical exercise, cognitive exercise, stress, and depression. I was pleasantly surprised and intrigued because I have seen firsthand the importance of a healthy lifestyle in addition to medicines in treating dementia. I was curious about how she planned on implementing these interventions. Never before had I seen such an integrated approach organized in this way. Dr. Vojtkofsky offered to provide me with the research that backs up these interventions.

I said, "Stop right there. I know exactly what you are talking about. I've seen the research, and seen results of treatment like this directly in my patients. Those who implement lifestyle changes—and exercise their brain—have a better trajectory for their illness than patients who don't."

Keep Your Brain Stronger for Longer has suitable cognitive exercises that are specifically tailored for people with MCI. I love that it includes exercises for all cognitive abilities, not just memory; the usual complaint of people with mild cognitive impairment (MCI). They often think that memory is their only problem and neglect other important brain abilities, like language and reasoning, which need exercising too. *Keep Your Brain Stronger for Longer* has practical exercises designed to strengthen and maintain functional abilities that begin to decline in MCI, like calendar scheduling, time telling, and calculation skills needed for everyday activities. Each page tells the reader which cognitive ability they are exercising to educate them on how to decipher the differences between cognitive abilities. Readers are implicitly learning about their brains along the way. This book assuredly promotes brain health and empowers people to have influence over their cognitive future, serving them, their families, and society in general.

I was impressed by Dr. Vojtkofsky's innovation at that first meeting, but more I was relieved to know someone was finally providing this service in my community. I would now have a place to refer my patients with MCI and mild dementia where they will get education and support on how to keep their brains stronger for longer. And not just in words, but in actions.

Cognitive Care Solutions offers a lifestyle action plan: In sessions, the therapists actually exercise clients' brains and provide other psychological interventions. They can show my patients, their families, and me significant results through serial neuropsychological testing.

After just meeting Dr. Vojtkofsky and talking for about twenty minutes, I proceeded to offer her company a space in my clinical trial research office to see patients. Now we are colleagues working side by side to provide dementia patients and their families empowerment to reach their highest health potential. No, we can't cure this disease, but we definitely can treat it and improve individuals' and their caregivers' quality of life.

ROBERT G. FELDMAN, MD, is the founder and Medical Director of Senior Clinical Trials, Inc., a private practitioner in Laguna Hills, California, and a member of the Medical Science Advisory Board of the Orange County Alzheimer's Association.

INTRODUCTION

A Well-Rounded Workout for the Brain

THE GREATEST FEAR among older adults is dementia, and mild cognitive impairment (MCI) is a large risk factor for dementia. Today six million people in the United States have MCI, and 7 percent of older adults develop it every year.

As a doctor of psychology specializing in Alzheimer's disease and related dementias, I am often asked by seniors in the community, "How can I reduce my risk for dementia?," and by those with MCI, "What can I do to stay strong?"

My answer is always: Exercise your brain! Research has shown the benefits of keeping cognitive abilities strong. Those who have challenged their brains throughout their life have a lower risk of developing dementia,* and those who have MCI and exercise their brains can keep their cognitive abilities stronger for longer.†

This workbook has been specifically designed to help those with MCI exercise their brain. It provides a variety of exercises for different cognitive abilities. Research supports that brain exercise 1) must be challenging, and 2) must target various cognitive abilities, not just one (e.g., only doing crossword puzzles).

When I started my private practice, I searched for curriculum at all ability levels and found little to nothing for impaired adults. Most of the brain exercise workbooks are for healthy adults with no impairment, which is too difficult for my clients. I could not find curriculum at the difficulty level of MCI that was appropriate for adults; they all had children's animation and topics of interest for kids. I refused to give my respectable clients worksheets for kids, as I felt it was pejorative to their dignity. I got so angry at the amount of time I was spending reformatting other people's curriculum that I decided to write my own cognitive exercise book for adults with MCI, with topics they would find interesting. So this book is my gift to you. I hope you enjoy using it as much as I have enjoyed developing it for you.

Our brains need a well-rounded workout just like our bodies!

In this workbook, each worksheet is labeled with the cognitive ability that is being exercised. Since many of the tasks exercise multiple cognitive abilities, I have labeled the worksheet with the primary cognitive ability the task targets.

There is no one right way to approach this book. You can start at the beginning and work your way through the exercises in order, or you can pick and choose the abilities you would like to work on each day.

I do recommend that you complete a variety of exercises targeting different cognitive abilities in each sitting, which is the best way to get a well-rounded workout. Just like our bodies, if we only lifted weights for one muscle and not all the others, it would not be a very good workout. I also recommend doing a minimum of three hours per week of cognitive exercise. The American Medical Association recommends a minimum of three hours per week of physical exercise, and I believe we should do the same for the brain.

As you work your way through this book, you might notice that there are many more language exercises than other targeted cognitive ability tasks, such as memory. Yes, this was intentional. In case you are wondering, here's the reason why: Usually people with MCI struggle the most with short-term memory. I wanted to exercise memory in a simple way, but not overdo it, so that you wouldn't become discouraged and quit if you had to struggle through many of the exercises. Language, on the other hand, is an ability that is still relatively strong in people with MCI. We want to exercise it a lot so that it stays strong for as long as possible. Many people with MCI will have that "tip-of-the-tongue" phenomenon in which they cannot think of words as quickly as before. These many language exercises will help you strengthen those neural networks and potentially increase word retrieval speed. Other cognitive abilities have even fewer exercises, such as attention and sequencing, because those cognitive abilities are being exercised in many of the other tasks, but are secondary to the one listed on the page.

All of the exercises require attention, and many require sequencing, but neither is often listed as the "primary" cognitive ability being targeted.

What this workbook is *not*

This workbook is not intended to cure or reverse your MCI. This workbook is intended to exercise your brain and keep you mentally stimulated with a variety of different tasks. My goal is to keep your brain stronger for longer. Now let's have some fun!

---

* Verghese et al. (2003). Leisure activities and the risk of dementia in the elderly. *New England Journal of Medicine*, 348(25), 2508–16.

† Reijnders et al. (2013). Cognitive interventions in healthy older adults and people with mild cognitive impairment: A systematic review. *Aging Resources Review*, 12(1), 263–75.

COGNITIVE ABILITIES

A Quick Reference Guide

ATTENTION is a state of awareness in which the senses are focused exclusively on a particular aspect of the environment.

CALCULATION is the ability to compute numbers using mathematical operations such as addition, subtraction, multiplication, or division.

EXECUTIVE FUNCTIONING is a set of mental processes that help people perform activities such as planning, organizing, sequencing, and set-shifting.

LANGUAGE is the ability to use a system of letters and words to express ideas and communicate.

MEMORY is the ability to input, store, and retrieve information.

PROCESSING SPEED is a measure of cognitive efficiency, that is, it is the ability to process information quickly (i.e., mental movement from one item to the next).

REASONING is the ability to think in a logical way, moving step-by-step to form a conclusion.

SEQUENCING is the ability to arrange items in a particular requested order.

VISUAL-SPATIAL SKILL is an ability to understand visual stimuli and the spatial relationships of objects. It allows people to maneuver through space, such as finding their car in a parking lot, and using a map.

TO DO AND REMEMBER, FOR A SUCCESSFUL WORKOUT

1. Keep your body and your mind relaxed.

Your brain works best when you are relaxed. If you find yourself getting stressed out, push the workbook aside and take a few deep breaths and focus on relaxing your body, and then your mind will follow. When ready, go back to the exercise.

2. Everybody makes mistakes.

No one is perfect. Therefore, I recommend you use a pencil to complete these exercises and have plenty of erasers handy. It is easier to correct pencil marks than pen.

3. Keep trying.

The benefit of cognitive exercise is when something is challenging but you keep trying to figure it out. If every task was easy, then you would not get to strengthen your brain. If needed, skip a tough task and come back to it later. Unaware to you, the brain will work on it, and when you go back the answer might just pop out at you.

4. Don't criticize yourself.

You are trying your best and there is no shame in that, so you are not allowed to judge or criticize yourself for getting a wrong answer or not being able to complete a task. *No one* will get every answer in this workbook correct on the first try. If you are absolutely lost on what the answer is, go look it up in the answer section at the back of the workbook. Then go back and figure out *why* that is the right answer. That reasoning process will help you understand, and that kind of learning strengthens the brain!

KEEP YOUR
BRAIN
STRONGER
FOR
LONGER

THE
EXERCISES

GRANDCHILDREN COMPARISONS

Using the clues given, make the requested comparisons to determine the correct answer.

1. Your grandchildren are racing in the backyard. Jimmy beat Cathy, and Melanie beat Patrick. If Patrick beat Jimmy, what was the outcome of the race?

1ST PLACE	
2ND PLACE	
3RD PLACE	
4TH PLACE	

2. Your grandchildren are measuring their heights. Tom is taller than Sally, but he is not taller than Lucy. Amber is not as tall as Sally. What is their order of height from tallest to shortest?

1ST (TALLEST)	
2ND	
3RD	
4TH (SHORTEST)	

3. Your grandchildren are comparing their allowances. Kate earns more than Henry, who earns the least. Joe does not make as much as Kate. What is their order from the highest allowance to the least?

1ST (HIGHEST)	
2ND	
3RD (LEAST)	

REASONING

4. Your grandchildren are comparing their grades. Yvonne earned a higher grade than Albert, but she did not earn as high of a grade as Neil. Marie earned a higher grade than Neil. What is their order from highest grade to lowest grade?

1ST (HIGHEST)	
2ND	
3RD	
4TH (LOWEST)	

5. Your grandchildren are comparing how many toys they have at your house. Louie has less than Tamra, who has less than Olivia. Robert has more toys than Olivia. What is their order from the most toys to the least?

1ST (MOST)	
2ND	
3RD	
4TH (LEAST)	

6. Your grandchildren are playing a board game. Eva has 4 more points than William, but she has 8 less points than Vivian. If William has 32 points, in what order did they come in the game and with how many points?

	NAME	POINTS
1ST		
2ND		
3RD		

TWO DEFINITIONS 1

Two definitions for the same word are given. Fill in the correct word that matches both definitions.

1. To fight with your fists

   A container

   ANSWER _____

2. Area with no sun

   A tint of color

   ANSWER _____

3. Part of a tree

   A large suitcase

   ANSWER _____

4. Smart

   Sunny

   ANSWER _____

5. A measurement

   Part of the body

   ANSWER _____

6. A stone

   To sway back and forth

   ANSWER _____

7. To hit with a fist

   A fruit drink

   ANSWER _____

8. To say clearly

   Temperament

   ANSWER _____

MATCHING CLUES 1

Match two of the word-parts to make a word that fits the clue. Each word-part is used only once.

je	jo	re	int
bel	jo	wel	ban

1. _____ a stringed musical instrument

   _____ to rise in opposition

   _____ a precious stone

   _____ where two parts fit together

aj	ck	jo	ar
ke	ke	ba	ba

2. _____ a punch line

   _____ slightly open

   _____ to cook with dry heat

   _____ toward the rear

SEQUENCING ITEMS 1

Discover a logical way to sequence these items, and explain the *reason* why you put them in that order. No alphabetical order allowed. There may be more than one correct answer.

1. Flea, Bumblebee, Ladybug, Butterfly

   1st _____ 2nd _____ 3rd _____ 4th _____

   Reason _____

2. Semester, Month, Centennial, Fiscal year

   1st _____ 2nd _____ 3rd _____ 4th _____

   Reason _____

3. Paint, Chop, Carve, Sand

   1st _____ 2nd _____ 3rd _____ 4th _____

   Reason _____

4. Millimeter, Kilometer, Meter, Centimeter

   1st _____ 2nd _____ 3rd _____ 4th _____

   Reason _____

5. Mortgage, Escrow, Credit check pre-approval, Offer

   1st _____ 2nd _____ 3rd _____ 4th _____

   Reason _____

6. Check mirrors, Press gas pedal, Put into drive, Fasten seat belt

   1st _____ 2nd _____ 3rd _____ 4th _____

   Reason _____

7. Bake, Gather ingredients, Mix, Pour into pan

   1st _____ 2nd _____ 3rd _____ 4th _____

   Reason _____

8. Hill, Pebble, Mountain, Boulder

1st _____ 2nd _____ 3rd _____ 4th _____

Reason _____

9. Large intestine, Small intestine, Mouth, Stomach

1st _____ 2nd _____ 3rd _____ 4th _____

Reason _____

10. Cocoon, Butterfly, Caterpillar, Egg

1st _____ 2nd _____ 3rd _____ 4th _____

Reason _____

11. Night, Dawn, High noon, Dusk

1st _____ 2nd _____ 3rd _____ 4th _____

Reason _____

12. Nose, Blood, Body tissue, Lungs

1st _____ 2nd _____ 3rd _____ 4th _____

Reason _____

13. Bacteria, Cow, Yogurt, Milk

1st _____ 2nd _____ 3rd _____ 4th _____

Reason _____

14. Application, Attendance, Acceptance, Interview

1st _____ 2nd _____ 3rd _____ 4th _____

Reason _____

15. Hypothesis, Results, Experiment, Analysis

1st _____ 2nd _____ 3rd _____ 4th _____

Reason _____

FAMILY TREE GAME 1

Based on this family tree, answer the questions below with a specific name.

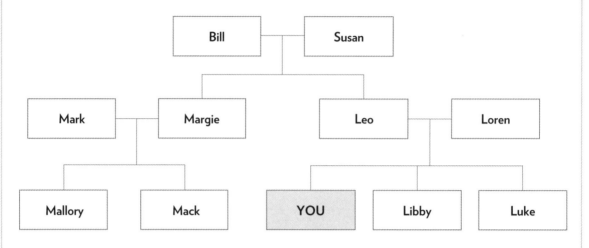

1. Who is your father's father's son?

   _____

2. Who is your mother's husband's mother?

   _____

3. Who is your uncle's daughter?

   _____

4. Who are your cousins?

   _____

5. Who is your aunt's husband?

   _____

6. Who is your grandfather's daughter-in-law?

   _____

REASONING

BOXED LETTERS – CARDS

Print the letters in the correct box to spell a type of card game reading across.

1. Print the letter O in box B2
Print the letter H in box D6
Print the letter I in box A4
Print the letter F in box C3
Print the letter S in box B5
Print the letter G in box C1

ANSWER _____

	1	2	3	4	5	6
A						
B						
C						
D						

2. Print the letter K in box C3
Print the letter R in box D5
Print the letter E in box A4
Print the letter P in box B1
Print the letter O in Box A2

ANSWER _____

	1	2	3	4	5	6	7	8	9
A									
B									
C									
D									

3. Print the letter A in A3
Print the letter S in C6
Print the letter E in D2
Print the letter T in B5
Print the letter H in B1
Print the letter R in C4   ANSWER _____

	1	2	3	4	5	6
A						
B						
C						
D						

4. Print the letter M in B6
Print the letter N in C3
Print the letter U in A5
Print the letter I in D2
Print the letter Y in C8
Print the letter G in B1
Print the letter M in A7
Print the letter R in D4   ANSWER _____

	1	2	3	4	5	6	7	8
A								
B								
C								
D								

VISUAL-SPATIAL

5. Print the letter A in B3
Print the letter S in C6
Print the letter P in C2
Print the letter E in D5
Print the letter S in B1
Print the letter D in A4　　　　　　　　ANSWER _____

	1	2	3	4	5	6
A						
B						
C						
D						

6. Print the letter I in box B7
Print the letter A in box C3
Print the letter Y in box D5
Print the letter H in box A9
Print the letter R in box C2
Print the letter S in box C11
Print the letter G in box A8
Print the letter C in box D1
Print the letter E in Box B6
Print the letter Z in Box C4
Print the letter T in Box A10　　　　　　ANSWER _____

	1	2	3	4	5	6	7	8	9	10	11
A											
B											
C											
D											

TWO-LETTER PLACEMENT 1

Choose which two-letter combo will make a word when added to the letters below. There may be more than one possible answer.

er   ar   or   to   se   re   ra

1. o d __ __

2. a d h __ __ e

3. b __ __ w

4. f __ __ m

5. d r e __ __ y

6. a v __ __ a g e

7. c a __ __

8. h __ __ d

9. c o t __ __ n

10. p l u __ __ l

11. s h __ __ t

12. c a r e __ __

13. s p __ __ y

14. o r c h __ __ d

15. s e c __ __ t

16. s __ __ r e

17. p a __ __ n t

18. __ __ g u e

19. g __ __ e d

20. e __ __ l y

21. c o __ __ c e

22. m __ __ g i n a l

23. __ __ i g i n

24. g u __ __ d

25. i n __ __ r t

26. a v __ __ s i o n

27. c l o __ __ t

28. s c __ __ n

29. l a p __ __ p

30. t h __ __ a d

31. c __ __ a m i c

32. __ __ a s t

33. e r a __ __

34. c __ __ k

LANGUAGE

DECIPHER THE LETTER CODE 1

Complete the phrase by determining the number that is assigned to the used letters.

Begin by filling in the letters that you are given, then figure out which letters make sense to make words in the phrase. You don't have to figure out all the letters, just the ones you need.

For example, if the word is ____ H̲ ____ , the word is likely THE, so 8 = T,
　　　　　　　　　　　　　8　　13

therefore you can add in all 8's as T's.

A	B	C	D	E	F	G	H	I	J	K	L	M
10		3		7		1	24					

N	O	P	Q	R	S	T	U	V	W	X	Y	Z
25						2			5		15	

MESSAGE:

5 24 7 25   7 19 7 9 15 2 24 18 25 1   18 23

3 12 14 18 25 1   15 12 8 9   5 10 15 ,

15 12 8   10 9 7   18 25   2 24 7

5 9 12 25 1   22 10 25 7 .

WHAT'S THAT PHRASE? 1

Fill in the letters to complete the familiar phrase. There is a clue to help.

1. A D ___ ___ ___   A D ___ ___ ___ ___

When something is extremely common

2. A P ___ ___ ___ ___   O ___   C ___ ___ ___

A task that is simple to complete

3. A ___ ___   A ___ ___ ___   A ___ ___   A L ___ ___ ___

When something is extremely expensive, it costs . . .

4. I ___ ' ___   A ___ ___   G ___ ___ ___ ___ ___   T ___   M ___ ___

When something is incomprehensible

5. B ___ ___ ___ ___   T ___ ___   T ___ ___ ___   D ___ ___   W ___ ___ ___ ___

B ___ ___ ___ ___ D

To start over again after a failed attempt is to go . . .

6. B ___ ___ ___   T   A ___ ___ ___ ___ ___   D T ___ ___ ___   B ___ ___ ___ ___ ___

When someone avoids the main point or fails to get to the bottom line

7. B ___ ___   W ___ ___ ___ ___   A R ___ ___ K A ___ ___ ___   A

H ___ ___ D P ___ ___ ___ ___ E

When someone is faced with two difficult decisions; a dilemma

8. B ___ ___ ___ ___ ___ K T ___ ___ ___   I ___ ___ ___

To end the social awkwardness

9. B ___ ___ ___ ___ ___ ___ T Y ___ ___ R B ___ ___ ___   B ___ ___

To ruin someone's happy mood

MEMORY

10. C ___ ___ ___ E   B ___ ___   N ___   C ___ ___ ___ ___

To almost reach a successful outcome only to fall short at the end

11. C ___ ___   T ___   T ___ ___   C ___ ___ ___ E

To get to the point

12. D ___ ___   N   F ___ ___   T ___ ___   C ___ ___ ___ T

To look defeated or beaten

13. D ___ ___ ___   T ___   T ___ ___   W ___ ___ ___

When an outcome is determined in the last few seconds

14. D ___ ___   P ___ ___ ___ ___ ___   L ___ ___ ___   F ___ ___ ___ S

To fall down in large numbers

15. E ___ ___ ___   A ___   P ___ ___

Something that is simple

16. E ___ ___ ___ ___ ___ ___ ___   T   I ___   T ___ ___   R ___ ___ ___

The large obvious problem that is being ignored

COUNT THE U'S

As quickly as you can, count how many U's are in this paragraph. Scan each line from left to right.

a u l k d j f i s o d j h u i n d t u t y o e y k f s l y l k j l d f u i n f k s l l

w o q p o w r y r j k u l y s k d n f k s l u k s d n f u k j f k s d n f u n s k

d f n d l u k s d n f s k d u n k l p u n s d l f y a d f u l j u p i u w e r u p

o u w e r u l s u e r u l s i u s l d i u z m c v u z n u d n f u e r y u s d l k

f u u n l s u p i u r q w e u l s d f u l k j u l k u k l f s d i f u s d f u x c v

m n d f u s w e r u r y u x g u a d f g u l k j u o i u w e r u s d f u t w e r

u q w e u u u p o i u q w u a d f u z c v u m b n u k l j h s d f x c v i o s e

r k j a s d y s d f o l u n k e r j u s d f u w e r t w e m x g p q w i u y s d f

j n k u y t w e r l k d f u q w e r u x c b h s d f g b z v x c y t w e r u u s

e b f s u y g e w u a o d p e y x o s d i u d s w x p o t h d k b s k o e r t n

v u e r b n l d k f y u l s k d u s h s e t u t u s k d o u d t h k s d u

TOTAL U'S _____

ATTENTION

AGING WORDS 1

The answer to each clue contains the letters "AGE."

1. A metal enclosure for confining animals

   ANSWER _CAGE_

2. A system of words to express thoughts

   ANSWER _LANGUAGE_

3. A connective protein found in skin

   ANSWER _COLLAGEN_

4. A restaurant fee for serving wine brought in from elsewhere

   ANSWER _CORKAGE_

5. A physical obstruction

   ANSWER _BLOCKAGE_

6. A small rural house situated in the countryside

   ANSWER _COTTAGE_

7. Discarded waste

   ANSWER _GARBAGE_

8. Something that passes from one generation to the next

   ANSWER _HERITAGE_

DOMINO ORDER 1

Starting with the domino marked "1st," find an order in which you can line up all these dominoes end to end. Wherever two dominoes touch, the numbered ends must match. You may rotate the dominoes, and there is more than one correct order.

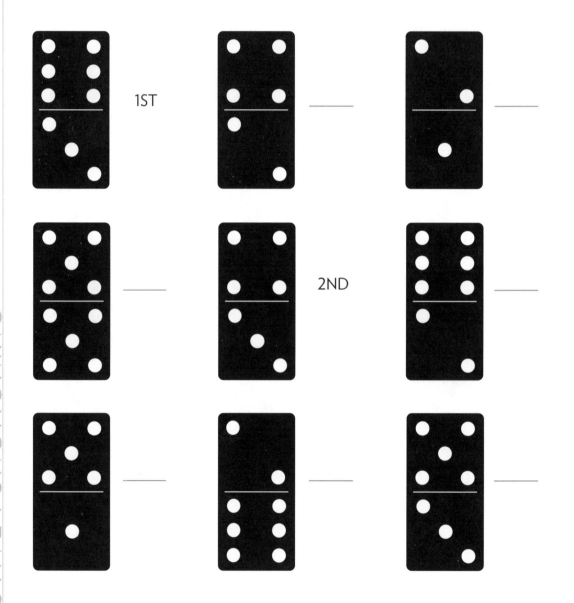

VENN DIAGRAM – LANGUAGES

Answer the questions using the information displayed in the Venn diagram.

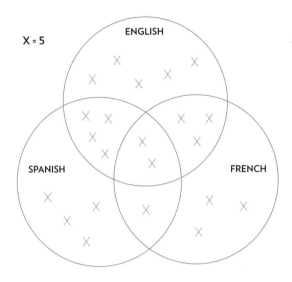

1. How many people speak only English and Spanish?

    ANSWER _____

2. Is it more common for people to speak all three languages or just Spanish and French?

    ANSWER _____

3. How many people speak only Spanish and French?

    ANSWER _____

4. How many people speak English?

    ANSWER _____

5. How many people speak only English?

    ANSWER _____

6. How many people do not speak French?

    ANSWER _____

DOT COPY 1

Copy these patterns onto the blank graphs.

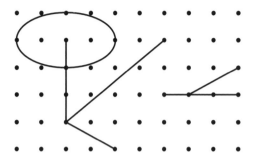
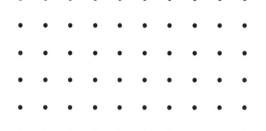

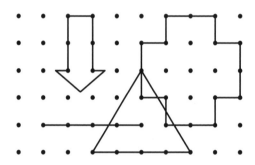
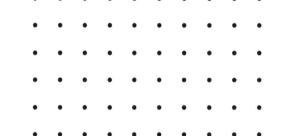

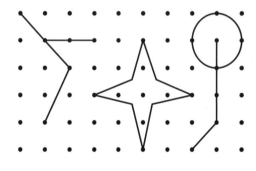

VISUAL–SPATIAL

SHAPE MATCH 1

Circle the two matching shapes.

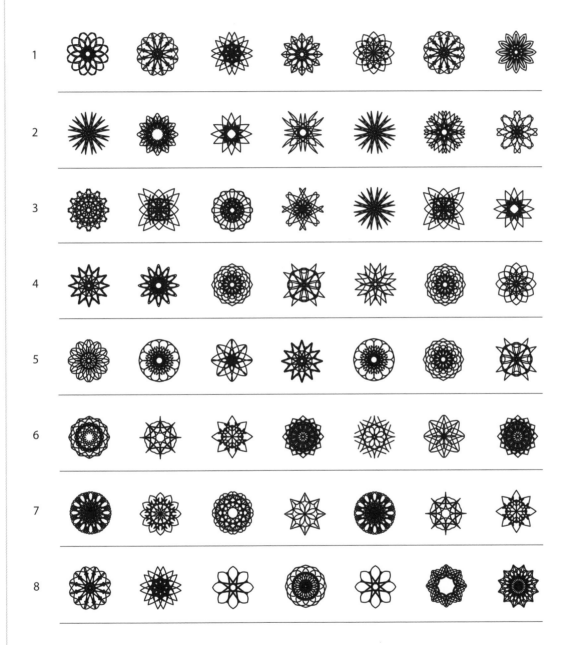

VISUAL–SPATIAL

LETTER TRANSFER 1

Fill in the word to answer the clue, then transfer those numbered letters to the lines below for the final message.

1. The instrument Miles Davis, the jazz musician, played

   ___ ___ ___ ___ ___ ___ ___
   1   2   3   4   5   6   1

2. This country has the most people

   ___ ___ ___ ___ ___
   8   9   10 11 12

3. The largest state in the United States

   ___ ___ ___ ___ ___ ___
   12 13 12 14 15 12

4. This indoor sport is the most popular in the United States

   ___ ___ ___ ___ ___ ___ ___ ___ ___ ___
   16 12 14 15 6   1   16 12 13 13

5. The Beatles recorded this album the last time they were together

   ___ ___ ___ ___ ___   ___ ___ ___ ___
   12 16 16 6   17   2   18 12 19

6. The largest mammal in the world

   ___ ___ ___ ___ ___
   22 9   12 13 6

7. A young delinquent is called this

   ___ ___ ___ ___ ___ ___ ___ ___
   23 3   24 6   11 10 13 6

FINAL MESSAGE:

___ ___ ___ ___ ___ ___   ___ ___ ___   ___ ___ ___ ___ ___   ___ ___ ___
12 13 22 12 17 14   2   6   4   6   4   16 6   2   17 18 3

___ ___ ___   ___ ___ ___ q___ ___ ,   ___ ___ ___ ___   ___ ___ ___ ___
12 2   6   3   11 10   3   6   23 3   14 1   13 10 15 6

___ ___ ___ ___ ___ ___ ___ ___ ___   ___ ___ ___ ___ .
6   24 6   2   17 16 18 19 17   6   13 14 6

CODING – FAMILY

Use the key code below to decode the words. Each space is one letter. Challenge yourself to go as quickly as you can. All of these words are in the category: **FAMILY**.

1.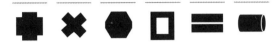

2.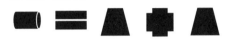

3.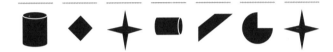

4.

5.

KEY CODE

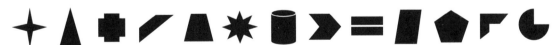

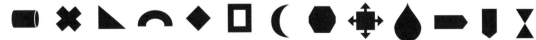

MATCHING CLUES 2

Match two of the word-parts to make a word that fits the clue. Each word-part is used only once.

ot   ree   deg   ru

sir   tar   de   en

1. _____   a fortune-teller's cards

   _____   a temperature unit

   _____   a warning horn

   _____   unmannerly

st   la   ra   ep

re   rp   te   ta

2. _____   not common

   _____   a stair

   _____   a canvas cover

   _____   tardy

FIRST AND LAST LETTERS 1

Fill in the correct letters to make a word that matches the definition.

1. ____ rat ____   a wooden box

2. ____ estor ____   to renovate

3. ____ res ____   a printing machine

4. ____ ton ____   to make amends

5. ____ ddres ____   a house location

6. ____ ee ____   a fruit rind

7. ____ nti ____   to loosen laces

8. ____ ot ____   a musical tone

9. ____ em ____   a floor model

10. ____ hee ____   transparent

11. ____ va ____   egg-shaped

12. ____ ria ____   a courtroom event

WORD MAZE – A LAZY SUNDAY

Find your way through the maze by connecting letters to spell out words.
Write the words on the next page. You may move right, left, up, or down, but no letters may be connected more than once.

START

A	P	T	R	W	Q	N	L	M	E	R	C
D	M	C	B	F	V	E	Y	K	P	D	O
G	N	O	L	S	E	W	S	P	A	H	F
W	H	K	J	R	H	X	T	H	L	E	F
A	L	K	Y	E	B	L	Y	O	D	E	Y
H	R	B	P	P	C	H	M	N	K	D	R
L	W	I	I	L	S	S	T	U	W	H	V
Q	Q	G	M	E	Q	L	K	A	C	B	Q
J	R	C	P	A	L	F	P	M	U	Y	P
O	L	N	B	V	F	A	C	B	S	O	T
M	A	S	D	B	A	M	U	P	V	B	N
B	K	P	B	I	M	B	C	K	N	F	B
G	J	C	Y	L	U	V	V	V	K	L	V

END

WORDS

1. _____

2. _____

3. _____

4. _____

5. _____

6. _____

7. _____

8. _____

9. _____

LOGIC WORD PROBLEMS 1

These word problems require you to use the process of elimination to find the answer. It helps to use the grid provided to keep track of items eliminated.

X = No, not the correct answer; O = Yes, the correct answer

Using the clues, fill in the grid with X's and O's. When there is only one choice left in a row or column, put an O there. Because it is the only option left, it is the correct answer. If a clue tells you the correct choice, you can put an O in that box and put X's in the rest of the column and row because the other options cannot be correct too. Work through all of the clues this way.

1. You take your 4 grandchildren to the pet store to pick out one pet each. Can you determine which grandchild picked out which pet?

	CAT	DOG	FISH	GERBIL
BILLY				
SALLY				
CATHY				
JOHN				

CLUES
a. John chose the pet that lives in the water.
b. Cathy did not choose the pet that starts with the same letter as her name.
c. Billy is allergic to cats but not to dogs
d. Cathy wants a pet that will live in a cage.

2. At a picnic each of your friends picked a different piece of fruit for dessert. Can you determine which friend picked which fruit?

	APPLE	ORANGE	BANANA	GRAPES
IRMA				
BETTY				
RALPH				
JIM				

CLUES
a. Betty grabbed a handful of her fruit and some fell and bounced around on the ground.
b. Ralph makes a joke about slipping on Irma's peel.
c. As he ate his fruit Jim said: "Eat one of these a day to keep the doctor away."

REASONING

MIDDLE LETTERS 1

Fill in the correct letters to make a word that matches the definition.

1. a _____ _____ m   a minute particle

2. o _____ _____ _____ r   external

3. a _____ _____ _____ e   to concur

4. a _____ _____ _____ a   a sports location

5. d _____ _____ t   a small arrow

6. a _____ _____ _____ e   unaccompanied

7. s _____ _____ _____ p   to use a broom

8. a _____ _____ _____ a   fragrance

9. s _____ _____ _____ t   slumbered

10. o _____ _____ n   plow-pulling animals

11. v _____ _____ _____ e   worth

12. s _____ _____ _____ e   a fixed gaze

BAGS OF WORDS

The answer to each clue contains the letters "BAG."

1. A ring-shaped bread roll

   ANSWER _____

2. A vehicle safety device

   ANSWER _____

3. A long thin loaf of French bread

   ANSWER _____

4. Another word for a purse

   ANSWER _____

5. A talkative person who has little of interest or value to say

   ANSWER _____

6. A large cushion used as a seat

   ANSWER _____

7. A vegetable with a leafy head

   ANSWER _____

8. A pouch attached to a horse or motorcycle

   ANSWER _____

LANGUAGE

ALLITERATION – PEOPLE

Alliteration is when all the words start with the same sound. Complete these sentences with words that begin with the same letter. You can add articles (such as *a, an, the*) or prepositions (such as *with, on, as*) to help the sentence make sense.

For example: Many moms making milkshakes.

1. Lawyers lurch_____.

2. Busy burglars_____.

3. _____ pilots play.

4. _____ seamstresses sewing.

5. Merry maids _____.

6. Vertical ventriloquists _____.

7. Parents purchasing _____.

8. Fickle females _____.

9. Pleasant professors _____.

10. Senseless stewardesses _____.

11. Matchmakers make _____.

12. _____ rise rapidly.

13. Architects' adversaries are _____.

14. Engineers' education _____.

15. _____ nurses nurturing.

TRUE OR FALSE FACTS 1

Determine if each statement is True or False. Challenge yourself to answer as quickly as you can.

1. An elephant is larger than a tiger. — True / False
2. Grape juice is darker than red wine. — True / False
3. Healthy has more letters than particular. — True / False
4. Several means more than a couple. — True / False
5. Fifteen-year-olds can get a driver's license. — True / False
6. Gold is heavier than aluminum. — True / False
7. A car is more expensive than a plane. — True / False
8. Sirens are louder than bells. — True / False
9. Walnut shells are softer than egg shells. — True / False
10. All mushrooms are edible. — True / False
11. Knifes can cut through cloth. — True / False
12. Aluminum foil can go in the microwave. — True / False
13. Bears have less fur than birds. — True / False
14. Both marbles and dice roll evenly. — True / False
15. Eagles are faster than jets. — True / False
16. Feathers are not lighter than air — True / False
17. Pillows are softer than hay. — True / False

PROCESSING SPEED

18. Windshields shatter easier than plastic.   True   False

19. The word "screen" has more than one definition.   True   False

20. Rubber bands stretch easier than paper clips.   True   False

21. Orchestras never have a conductor.   True   False

22. Porcupines are larger than splinters.   True   False

23. Bulls are the same size as goats.   True   False

24. "Racecar" is the same when spelled backwards.   True   False

PROCESSING SPEED

SYMBOL CODING 1

Write the symbol that corresponds to each number in the empty boxes below. Challenge yourself to do this as quickly as you can, while maintaining accuracy. Do not do all of one symbol at a time. Complete each box in a row moving from left to right, and then continue to the next line.

KEY CODE

1	2	3	4	5	6	7	8	9
+	□	⇑	—	△	✕	○	⊔	◇

2	5	4	7	6	3	8	5	9	1
3	6	7	8	3	4	9	1	2	5
5	9	1	4	2	7	5	9	8	6
6	2	3	6	9	8	1	3	4	5
7	9	3	1	4	2	7	8	5	6
4	1	6	8	2	9	3	5	4	2
1	5	7	4	3	6	2	1	9	3
6	3	1	7	2	5	9	8	2	1

PROCESSING SPEED

LETTERS-TO-WORD MATCH 1

There are 10 six-letter words that have been broken into chunks of three letters. These chunks have been mixed up, no chunk is used twice, and all chunks are used.

Can you determine what the 10 words are?

den	mag	det	est
ier	har	cal	use
ent	ach	fin	dam
blo	acq	net	uit
mer	bus	par	sel

1. _____

2. _____

3. _____

4. _____

5. _____

6. _____

7. _____

8. _____

9. _____

10. _____

THREE-LETTER PLACEMENT 1

Choose which three-letter combination will make a word when added to the letters below. There may be more than one correct answer.

bic   sal   gan   tin   ren   fan   dar

1. r a ___ ___ ___

2. s l o ___ ___ ___

3. a e r o ___ ___ ___

4. f r o s ___ ___ ___ g

5. ___ ___ ___ t i n e

6. a p p a ___ ___ ___ t

7. ___ ___ ___ a t i c

8. i n s ___ ___ ___ c t

9. ___ ___ ___ y c l e

10. ___ ___ ___ k e n

11. ___ ___ ___ e s

12. r e v e ___ ___ ___ t

13. i n ___ ___ ___ t

14. a c c u ___ ___ ___

15. m a ___ ___ ___ e e

16. b o u n ___ ___ ___ y

17. e l e _____ _____ _____ t

18. _____ _____ _____ a d

19. a r r o _____ _____ _____ t

20. r e _____ _____ _____ a

21. _____ _____ _____ k e r

22. o r _____ _____ _____ i z e

23. _____ _____ _____ v a g e

24. _____ _____ _____ g l e

25. p r o _____ _____ _____ e

26. s t _____ _____ _____ g t h

27. _____ _____ _____ l i n g

28. c u _____ _____ _____ a l

29. o r _____ _____ _____

30. _____ _____ _____ c y

31. o u _____ _____ _____ g

32. _____ _____ _____ e p s

33. w _____ _____ _____ c h

34. _____ _____ _____ u t e

ONLY THREE CLUES

Use these clues to answer each question.

1. You store things here.

   It is in the bottom part of a house.

   Mice like to live here.

   What is the place? _____

2. Kids like to play here.

   It is outside.

   There are paths to walk on here.

   What is the place? _____

3. It is made of soft fabric.

   It comes in many colors and designs.

   You use it in the bathroom or at a swimming pool.

   What is the item? _____

4. It cleans your house.

   It has a motor.

   Most dogs are afraid of it.

   What is the item?_____

5. It can be made of glass or plastic.

   It holds liquid.

   Its shape is a long cylinder.

   What is the item? _____

WHAT'S THE CATEGORY? 1

Put these words into the most correct category.

cabinet handles   poison ivy   calculator   duct tape
ladder   printer   floor wax   slide
hikers   concrete mix   landmark   stamps
wall mounts   paper weight   to-do list   fire pit
strollers   books

1. Things found in a hardware store

------------------------------------ ------------------------------------

------------------------------------ ------------------------------------

------------------------------------ ------------------------------------

2. Things found in a park

------------------------------------ ------------------------------------

------------------------------------ ------------------------------------

------------------------------------ ------------------------------------

3. Things found in an office

------------------------------------ ------------------------------------

------------------------------------ ------------------------------------

------------------------------------ ------------------------------------

UNITS OF TIME 1

Determine the correct answer to each question. Try to do the math in your head first, then use scratch paper if needed. Do not use a calculator.

1. How many minutes are in 4 hours? _____

2. How many seconds are in 2 ½ hours? _____

3. How many hours do 120 minutes and 10,800 seconds equal?

    _____

4. In 8 hours, it will be 5:00 a.m. What time is it now? _____

5. In 14 hours, it will be 8:00 p.m. What time is it now? _____

6. In 4 ½ hours, you will be 30 minutes late for your 2:00 p.m. appointment.

    What time is it now? _____

7. You started doing yard work at 8:00 a.m. You spent 1 ½ hours weeding, 45 minutes planting seeds, 20 minutes watering, and then 15 minutes cleaning up.

    What time is it now? _____

8. You need to do all your errands before you meet friends for lunch at 12:30 p.m. First you need to go to the bank (20 minutes), pick up dry cleaning across town (35 minutes), buy household items at the store (45 minutes), return library books (15 minutes), and then pick up repaired jewelry (25 minutes).

    How long will it take you to do these errands? _____

    What time do you need to leave the house to get all of these errands completed? _____

9. You are flying from Denver to Seattle to visit you family for the summer. The morning of your flight, you hear that your plane is delayed 3 hours. You had a 1-hour layover midway, where you were supposed to change planes with the connection flight leaving at 11:00 a.m. You now have to change that connection flight.

   If you are now flying out of Denver at 9:30 a.m., which connection flight to Seattle can you catch?   a. 1:00 p.m. flight   b. 7:50 p.m. flight

10. Your walk around the neighborhood each day takes you 47 minutes. But today you stop to talk with Emma for 12 minutes, then you help Bruce pick up his trash can that fell overnight, and talk to him, for 7 minutes, then you help Lou look for his lost dog for 26 minutes, then Lynn calls you inside to taste her banana bread for 11 minutes, and then on the way home you stop and tell Emma all that happened for 4 minutes.

    How much total time were you out in the neighborhood today?
    _____

    If you left at 10:35 a.m., what time did you arrive back home?
    _____

11. You are cooking dinner for your family who arrives at 6:00 p.m. The meat needs to simmer for 40 minutes on the stove, the scalloped potatoes bake for 105 minutes in the oven, and the green beans will take 35 minutes on the stove. You will need 30 minutes of preparation time to get started.

    How much total time do you need to cook dinner? _____

    What time do you need to start cooking to serve dinner at 6:30 p.m.?
    _____

12. You live on the east coast and your daughter lives on the west coast. You want to call her after she gets off work at 5:00 p.m. but before she eats dinner at 7:00 p.m. You are 3 hours ahead of her time. What is the time frame you have to call her in your eastern standard time? _____

CALCULATION

"B" WORDS

Using two clues, fill in the correct word that begins with "B."

1. A bee does this

   Excited talk

   ANSWER _____

2. The wind does this

   To project

   ANSWER _____

3. To participate in this rough sport

   A cardboard carrier

   ANSWER _____

4. A horse does this

   A dollar

   ANSWER _____

5. To wax your car

   A muscular man is this

   ANSWER _____

6. Not the front

   Pain in your lower . . .

   ANSWER _____

7. A tied ribbon

   After a performance

   ANSWER _____

8. A short-legged omnivorous animal

   To pester someone

   ANSWER _____

9. To come together

   A group of instruments

   ANSWER _____

10. A wooden stick

    A winged animal

    ANSWER _____

11. A curve in the road

    To bow forward

    ANSWER _____

12. A color

    A feeling

    ANSWER _____

13. To load a boat

    A flat piece of wood

    ANSWER _____

14. A type of wine

    To show embarrassment

    ANSWER _____

LANGUAGE

15. To schedule a flight

Bound written sheets of paper

ANSWER _____

16. A crisp candy

Frail

ANSWER _____

17. To have no money

To snap into two pieces (past tense)

ANSWER _____

18. A lure

To deliberately taunt

ANSWER _____

WHAT IS THIS CALLED?

Use the clue to determine what is being described.

1. A wooden object used to hold up wet clothes to dry on a clothesline
   _____

2. A plush toy that children love to hug _____

3. Cheerleaders carry these in parades _____

4. This is made by stitching together squares of fabric and padding
   _____

5. A two-wheeled means of transportation _____

6. A petrified artifact found deep in the ground _____

7. These insects make a rhythmical chirping sound _____

8. This leisurely sport requires a line and pole _____

9. You win a game of chess with this final move _____

10. A plastic payment option _____

11. Skiing over flat, open terrain _____

12. Text of dialogue (subtitling) on a TV screen _____

DOMINO ORDER 2

Starting with the domino marked "1st," find an order in which you can line up all these dominoes end to end. Wherever two dominoes touch, the numbered ends must match. You may rotate the dominoes, and there is more than one correct order.

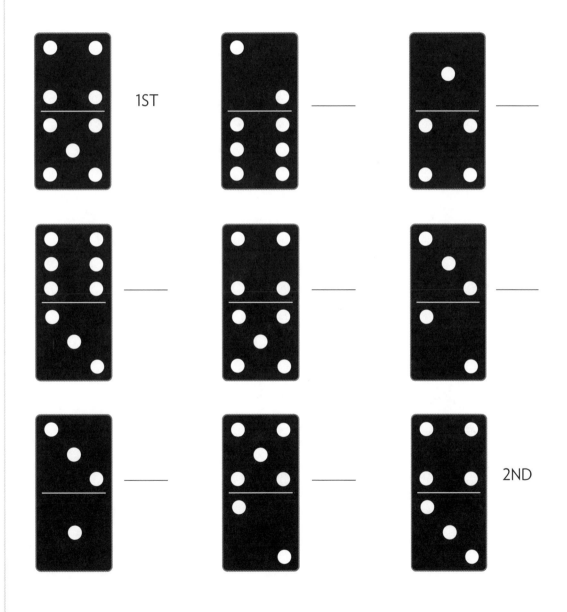

VENN DIAGRAM – BOOKS

Answer the questions using the information displayed in the Venn diagram.

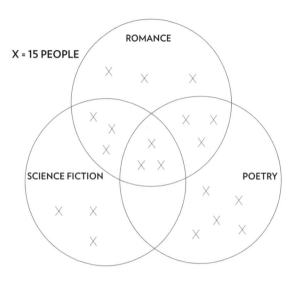

1. How many people like science fiction?

    ANSWER _____

2. Do more people like romance or poetry?

    ANSWER _____

3. How many people like only poetry and science fiction?

    ANSWER _____

4. How many people like poetry?

    ANSWER _____

5. How many people like only poetry?

    ANSWER _____

6. How many people do not like poetry?

    ANSWER _____

VISUAL–SPATIAL

DECIPHER THE LETTER CODE 2

Complete the phrase by determining the number that is assigned to the used letters.

Begin by filling in the letters that you are given, then figure out which letters make sense to make words in the phrase. You don't have to figure out all the letters, just the ones you need.

For example, if the word is ____ <u>H</u> ____ , the word is likely THE, so 8 = T,
                8   13

therefore you can add in all 8's as T's.

A	B	C	D	E	F	G	H	I	J	K	L	M
14	6						16				5	

N	O	P	Q	R	S	T	U	V	W	X	Y	Z
	15	4						17	9			

MESSAGE:

16　14　5　11　15　11　8　16　23　4　23　15　4　5　23

24　22　8　16　23　9　15　25　5　2　14　25　23

6　23　5　15　9　14　17　23　25　14　7　23 .

AGING WORDS 2

The answer to each clue contains the letters "AGE."

1. A loan agreement between borrower and lender

   ANSWER _____

2. To save something damaged for further use

   ANSWER _____

3. A quality of being brave

   ANSWER _____

4. The leaves of a plant or tree

   ANSWER _____

5. A legally recognized relationship

   ANSWER _____

6. An absence of something that is needed

   ANSWER _____

7. An organizer of a business

   ANSWER _____

8. Deliberate destruction

   ANSWER _____

LANGUAGE

COUNT THE T'S AND P'S

As quickly as you can, separately count how many T's and P's are in this paragraph. Scan each line from left to right. Keep a running tally of T's in your mind while keeping a running tally of P's separately. Do not do one letter at a time, try to do both at the same time.

a u l p d j f i s o d j h u i n d t u t y o e y k f s l y l k j l d p u i n f k s l l

w o q p o w r y t j k u l y s k d n f k t l u k s d n f u k p t k s d n f u n s p

d f n t l u k s d n f t k d u n k l p u n s d l f y a d f u l t u p i u w e r u p k

o u w e r u l s u e r u l s i u s l d i p z m c v u z n u d t f u e r y u s d l k

f u u n l s u p i u r q w e u l s d f u l p j u l k u t l f s d i f u s d t u x c v

m n d f t s w e r u r y u x g u a d t g u l k j p o i u w e r u s d f u t w e r

u q w e u u u p o i u q w u a d f u z c v u m b n u k l t h s d f x c v i o s e

r p j a s d y s d t o l u n k e r j u s d f u w e r t w e m x g p q w i u y s d f

j n k u y t w e r l k d f u q w e r u x c b h s d f g p z v x c y t w e r u u s

e b f s u y p e w u a o d p e y x o s d i u t s w x p o t h d k b s k o e r t n

TOTAL T'S _____

TOTAL P'S _____

MISMATCH 1

Pick out the one item that does not fit the category, and explain the *reason* why it does not fit.

1. Shoe, Grocery, Hardware, Tooth

   Mismatch item_____

   *Reason*_____

2. Goat, Horse, Eagle, Sheep

   Mismatch item_____

   *Reason*_____

3. Apple, Cauliflower, Carrot, Broccoli

   Mismatch item_____

   *Reason*_____

4. Elephant, Shark, Gorilla, Tiger

   Mismatch Item_____

   *Reason*_____

5. Turtle, Lizard, Parrot, Frog

   Mismatch item_____

   *Reason*_____

6. Coloring book, Legos, Building blocks, Tinkertoys

   Mismatch item_____

   *Reason*_____

7. Pencil, Eraser, Marker, Pen

   Mismatch item_____

   *Reason*_____

8. Soccer, Lacrosse, Volleyball, Golf

   Mismatch item_____

   *Reason*_____

EXECUTIVE FUNCTIONING

9. Initiate, Dissolve, Originate, Create

Mismatch item_____

*Reason*_____

10. Entry, Admission, Window, Door

Mismatch item_____

*Reason*_____

11. Being, Individual, Creature, Separate

Mismatch item_____

*Reason*_____

12. Various, Single, Only, Individual

Mismatch item_____

*Reason*_____

13. Pint, Cup, Ounce, Inch

Mismatch item_____

*Reason*_____

14. Vegetables, Rice, Pasta, Beans

Mismatch item_____

*Reason*_____

15. Skis, Boots, Snow, Resort

Mismatch item_____

*Reason*_____

16. Helicopters, Stars, Black holes, Planets

Mismatch item_____

*Reason*_____

SIMILAR PROPERTIES

What do these two things have in common?

1. A Fish and a Lizard _____

2. Water and Steam _____

3. A Tornado and an Earthquake _____

4. A Coconut and a Safe _____

5. A Paper clip and Tape _____

6. A Coupon and a Credit card _____

7. A Budget and a Path _____

8. Fall and Spring _____

9. A Goal and a Target _____

10. A Wreath and an Ornament _____

11. A Mushroom and a Mountain _____

12. Sunflowers and Celery _____

BOXED LETTERS – GAMES

Print the letters in the correct box to spell a type of board game reading across.

1. Print the letter O in B4
   Print the letter O in C6
   Print the letter O in A2
   Print the letter N in D3
   Print the letter P in B5
   Print the letter L in A7
   Print the letter M in C1
   Print the letter Y in B8   ANSWER _____

	1	2	3	4	5	6	7	8
A								
B								
C								
D								

2. Print the letter I in box B9
   Print the letter E in box C6
   Print the letter A in box D2
   Print the letter H in box A8
   Print the letter T in box C3
   Print the letter S in box A7
   Print the letter L in box B5
   Print the letter T in box D4
   Print the letter P in Box A10
   Print the letter B in Box B1   ANSWER _____

	1	2	3	4	5	6	7	8	9	10
A										
B										
C										
D										

3. Print the letter B in box B6
Print the letter A in box C4
Print the letter C in box A2
Print the letter L in box A7
Print the letter R in box C3
Print the letter E in box D8
Print the letter B in box B5
Print the letter S in box D1   ANSWER _____

	1	2	3	4	5	6	7	8
A								
B								
C								
D								

4. Print the letter S in box B5
Print the letter S in box C4
Print the letter E in box C3
Print the letter H in box D2
Print the letter C in box A1   ANSWER_____

	1	2	3	4	5	6	7	8
A								
B								
C								
D								

VISUAL-SPATIAL

5. Print the letter A in box B5
Print the letter A in box C3
Print the letter S in box A8
Print the letter H in box A2
Print the letter E in box C7
Print the letter R in box D4
Print the letter D in box B6
Print the letter C in box B1   ANSWER_____

	1	2	3	4	5	6	7	8
A								
B								
C								
D								

6. Print the letter R in box B9
Print the letter I in box C2
Print the letter T in box D4
Print the letter N in box A7
Print the letter O in box C6
Print the letter I in box B5
Print the letter C in box B3
Print the letter Y in box C10
Print the letter P in Box C1
Print the letter A in Box B8   ANSWER_____

	1	2	3	4	5	6	7	8	9	10
A										
B										
C										
D										

VISUAL-SPATIAL

LETTER TRANSFER 2

Fill in the word(s) to answer the clue, then transfer those numbered letters to the lines on the next page for the final message.

1. You get this color if you mix red and yellow

———— ———— ———— ———— ———— ————
  1   2   3   4   5   6

2. This document contains this sentence: "We hold these truths to be self-evident, that all men are created equal."

———— ———— ———— ———— ———— ———— ———— ———— ———— ———— ————   ———— ————
  7   6   8   9   3   2   3   10   11   1   4   1   12

———— ———— ———— ———— ———— ———— ———— ———— ———— ———— ————
 11   4   7   6   13   6   4   7   6   4   8   6

3. Philadelphia is the capital of this state

———— ———— ———— ———— ———— ———— ———— ———— ———— ———— ———— ————
 13   6   4   4   14   15   9   16   3   4   11   3

4. This American city is known as the home of jazz

———— ———— ————   ———— ———— ———— ———— ———— ———— ————
  4   6   17   1   2   9   6   3   4   14

5. This US company is the largest manufacturer of chocolate

———— ———— ———— ———— ———— ———— ———— ' ————
 18   6   2   14   18   6   15   14

6. This scientist discovered the theory of relativity

———— ———— ———— ———— ———— ———— ———— ————
  6   11   4   14   10   6   11   14

MEMORY

7. The Kentucky Derby takes place in this month

‾‾‾‾ ‾‾‾‾ ‾‾‾‾
19   3   15

FINAL MESSAGE:

‾‾‾ ‾‾‾ ‾‾‾ ‾‾‾   ‾‾‾ ‾‾‾   ‾‾‾ ‾‾‾ ‾‾‾ ‾‾‾ ‾‾‾   ‾‾‾ ‾‾‾
17 18 6   4   11 10   8   1   19 6   14   10 1

‾‾‾ ‾‾‾ ‾‾‾ u‾‾‾ ‾‾‾ ‾‾‾ , ‾‾‾ ‾‾‾ ‾‾‾ ‾‾‾   ‾‾‾ ‾‾‾ ‾‾‾ ‾‾‾ ‾‾‾ ‾‾‾
10 18 1   5   18 10   14 1   19 6   13 6   1   13 9   6

‾‾‾ ‾‾‾ ‾‾‾   ‾‾‾ ‾‾‾   ‾‾‾ ‾‾‾ ‾‾‾ ‾‾‾ ‾‾‾ ‾‾‾ ‾‾‾ .
14 10 1   13 3   10   4   1   10 18 11 4   5

PROFESSIONAL CHARACTERISTICS

Match the three top characteristics needed for each profession. You may only use each characteristics once.

creativity   ability to delegate   courage   inspired
articulate   logical   loyal   endurance
spontaneous   empathetic   thorough   confident

1. A CEO: _____   _____

    _____

2. An artist: _____   _____

    _____

3. A physician: _____   _____

    _____

4. A soldier: _____   _____

    _____

5. List any six characteristics you think are important for a person in the clergy.

    _____   _____

    _____   _____

    _____   _____

REASONING

CALCULATION WORD PROBLEMS 1

Determine the correct answer to each question. Try to do the math in your head first, then use scratch paper if needed. Do not use a calculator.

1. You are having 6 friends over for a dinner party. You and your spouse want to make individual desserts for everyone but you have only 5 individual baking cups. How many more do you need to buy?

   _____ baking cups

2. Your 4 grandchildren are at your house playing. You have a pack of 30 stickers for them to use in coloring books. How many stickers does each child get if you divide them up evenly? How many stickers are left over?

   _____ stickers each   _____ are left over

3. Your book club meets once per month and the next book is 580 pages. How many pages do you have to read each day to have it completed by your next meeting if this month has 30 days? _____ pages

4. Your large family of 18 people is coming to your house for the Christmas holiday. There are 7 kids and 11 adults. You all decide that you will spend only $20 on each kid, and half that amount on each adult for presents. How much total money will you spend on gifts this year for your family, not including your spouse? _____ dollars

5. You are sitting in your backyard watching the birds in the tree. You watch 6 birds fly away, and then 4 more land. Now you count 14 birds total. How many birds were there in the beginning? _____ birds

6. While doing some yard work, you realize you need a really long rope. You have one piece of rope that is 8 feet 3 inches, and another piece of rope that is 12 feet 9 inches. If you use both, what is the total length of rope you have to use? _____ feet   _____ inches

CALENDAR QUIZ 1

Use the calendar clues to determine the correct date.

SUNDAY	MONDAY	TUESDAY	WEDNESDAY	THURSDAY	FRIDAY	SATURDAY
		1	2	3	4	5
6	7	8	9	10	11	12
13	14	15	16	17	18	19
20	21	22	23	24	25	26
27	28	29	30			

1. This date is on the middle day of the week.

   It is not in the first or last week of the month.

   It is a single digit date.

   What is the date? _____

2. This date is on a weekend.

   It falls in the middle week of the month.

   It is not the 19th.

   What is the date? _____

EXECUTIVE FUNCTIONING

3. This date is between the 16th and the 23rd.

It is on a day that begins with a "T."

On this date there are only 8 more days of the month left.

What is the date?_____

4. This date is a double digit.

It is not in the last half of a week.

It's digits add up to 4.

It is not on a Sunday.

What is the date? _____

A BIT OF WORDS

The answer to each clue contains the letters "BIT."

1. The curved path of a celestial object

    ANSWER _____

2. A burrowing, plant-eating animal with long ears

    ANSWER _____

3. A regular tendency or practice

    ANSWER _____

4. An amount of money removed from an account

    ANSWER _____

5. To formally forbid a person from doing something

    ANSWER _____

6. A public display in an art gallery

    ANSWER _____

7. Based on random choice or whim, rather than reason

    ANSWER _____

8. To live in or occupy

    ANSWER _____

REASONING

WHAT COMES NEXT?

Determine what comes next in this sequence and then explain the reason why.

1. Red, Orange, Yellow, Green, _____

*Reason*_____

2. Do, Re, Mi, Fa, _____

*Reason*_____

3. Baron, Earl, Duke, Prince, _____

*Reason*_____

4. Day, Week, Month, Year, _____

*Reason*_____

5. City, County, State, Country, _____

*Reason*_____

6. Whisper, Talk, Yell, _____

*Reason*_____

7. Two pair, Three of a kind, Straight, Flush, _____

*Reason*_____

8. Finger, Knuckle, Wrist, Elbow, _____

*Reason*_____

9. Pawn, Knight, Bishop, Rook, _____

*Reason*_____

REASONING

PLACEMENT OF LETTERS 1

Use the letters on the left to turn the word-parts on the right into complete words. You can use each word-part only once.

1. ffu

   shi

   ctf

   pli

   olo

   fic

   nef

   fan

   ec _____ gy

   am _____ fy

   in _____ cy

   fa _____ on

   be _____ it

   ta _____ ul

   di _____ se

   of _____ er

2. cto

   fol

   ari

   ffl

   sti

   rfo

   sti

   lfi

   pe _____ rm

   cl _____ fy

   te _____ fy

   fa _____ ry

   un _____ ds

   go _____ ng

   wa _____ es

   ju _____ fy

3. ref   re _____ al

oug   en _____ ge

nan   ca _____ ul

lar   fo _____ ge

fus   en _____ ce

for   br _____ ht

aff   fi _____ ce

ota   tr _____ ic

4. shf   se _____ sh

rti   de _____ se

rba   wi _____ ul

fen   fa _____ sy

lfi   di _____ am

lpf   ce _____ fy

agr   ga _____ ge

nta   he _____ ul

ABBREVIATIONS AND ACRONYMS

What do these abbreviations and acronyms stand for?

1. Capt. _____

2. UN _____

3. ASSN _____

4. est. _____

5. GOP _____

6. AWOL _____

7. inc. _____

8. BA _____

9. cent. _____

10. kg _____

11. lb _____

12. DC _____

13. cc _____

14. ltd _____

15. mph _____

16. Col. _____

17. NATO _____

18. oz _____

19. St. _____

MEMORY

LETTERS-TO-WORD MATCH 2

There are 10 six-letter words that have been broken into chunks of three letters. These chunks have been mixed up, no chunk is used twice, and all chunks are used.

Can you determine what the 10 words are?

can	hew	ble	ics
bou	act	fac	act
tor	pic	ach	kle
ual	nce	mas	ive
cot	opy	cas	eth

1. _____

2. _____

3. _____

4. _____

5. _____

6. _____

7. _____

8. _____

9. _____

10. _____

A BAN IN WORDS

The answer to each clue contains the letters "BAN."

1. A robber or outlaw belonging to a gang

ANSWER _____

2. A hut or shelter at the beach

ANSWER _____

3. To break up a group

ANSWER _____

4. An elaborate and formal meal for many people

ANSWER _____

5. To give up completely; cease to support

ANSWER _____

6. An upright structure at the side of a staircase

ANSWER _____

7. Residential; or dull and ordinary

ANSWER _____

8. A stringed musical instrument with a long neck and rounded body

ANSWER _____

9. Lacking in originality

ANSWER _____

10. To send someone away from a place as an official punishment

ANSWER _____

LANGUAGE

SYMBOL CODING 2

Write the number that corresponds to each symbol in the empty boxes below. Challenge yourself to do this as quickly as you can, while maintaining accuracy. Do not do all of one symbol at a time, complete each box in a row moving from left to right, and then continue to the next line.

KEY CODE

₪	ϙ	‡	◈	ʔ	§	¥	ɣ	ɔ
2	6	4	7	3	1	5	9	8

ʔ	₪	§	‡	ϙ	ɔ	◈	ɣ	‡	¥
◈	ϙ	ɔ	¥	§	‡	ϙ	ʔ	ɔ	ɣ
§	ʔ	‡	ϙ	◈	₪	¥	§	₪	ϙ
‡	ɣ	¥	ɔ	‡	§	ʔ	ϙ	‡	◈
₪	ɔ	◈	₪	ʔ	ϙ	¥	§	ɣ	ʔ
ϙ	ʔ	₪	§	‡	◈	ɣ	ɔ	¥	₪
◈	‡	¥	ʔ	ɔ	ϙ	₪	ɔ	‡	§

UNITS OF TIME 2

Determine the correct answer to each question. Try to do the math in your head first, then use scratch paper if needed. Do not use a calculator.

1. How many minutes are in 14 hours? _____

2. How many seconds are in 5 hours and 15 minutes? _____

3. How many hours equal 45 minutes and 8,100 seconds? _____

4. In 30 hours, it will be 8:00 a.m. What time is it now? _____

5. In 15 hours, it will be 10:00 p.m. What time is it now? _____

6. In 4 hours, you will be 15 minutes late for your 11:00 a.m. appointment.

   What time is it now? _____

7. You started cooking at 3:20 p.m. for your 6:00 p.m. dinner party. You spent 58 minutes on the appetizer soup, 14 minutes chopping vegetables, 44 minutes stir-frying, 6 minutes setting the table, and then 12 minutes cleaning up.

   What time is it now? _____

   How much time do you have to spare before the dinner party?

   _____

8. Your son lives on the west coast and you live on the east coast. Both of you want to schedule a phone call when the grandkids will be there. He gives you some available times: Saturday from 10:00 a.m. to 2:00 p.m. or after dinner between 8:00 and 9:00 p.m. You go to bed at 10:00 p.m.

   What is the time frame you have to call your son's family in your eastern standard time? _____

CALCULATION

DECIPHER THE LETTER CODE 3

Complete the phrase by determining the number that is assigned to the used letters.

Begin by filling in the letters that you are given, then figure out which letters make sense to make words in the phrase. You don't have to figure out all the letters, just the ones you need.

For example, if the word is ____ H ____ , the word is likely THE, so 8 = T,
                  8   13
therefore you can add in all 8's as T's.

A	B	C	D	E	F	G	H	I	J	K	L	M
9						13	21				23	8

N	O	P	Q	R	S	T	U	V	W	X	Y	Z
2					22				24		16	

MESSAGE:

___ ___ ___ ___ ___ ___   ___ ___ ___   ___ ___   ___ ___ ___ ___
8   6   11   11   23   19   9   13   19   6   22   24   21   19   18

___ ___ ___ ___   ___ ___ ___   ___ ___ ___ ___ ___ ___
16   2   14   12   9   13   19   22   5   9   12   5   22

___ ___   ___ ___ ___ ___   ___ ___ ___ ___ ___ ___
5   2   22   21   2   24   9   12   2   14   18   11

___ ___ ___ ___   ___ ___ ___ ___ ___ ___ .
16   2   14   12   8   6   11   11   23   19

COUNT THE Y'S AND I'S

As quickly as you can, count how many y's and i's are in this paragraph. Scan each line from left to right. Keep a running tally of both letters together. Don't do one letter at a time.

a u l k d j f i s o d j h u i n d t u t y o e y k f s l y l k j l d f u i n f k s l l

w o q p o w r y r j k u l y s k d n f k s l u k s d n f u k j f k s d n f u n s k

d f n d l u k s d n f s k d u n k l p u n s d l f y a d f u l j u p i u w e r u p

o u w e r u l s u e r u l s i u s l d i u z m c v u z n u d n f u e r y u s d l k

f u u n l s u p i u r q w e u l s d f u l k j u l k u k l f s d i f u s d f u x c v

m n d f u s w e r u r y u x g u a d f g u l k j y o i u w e r u s d f u t w e r

u q w e u u u p o i u q w u a d f u z c v u m b n u y l j h s d f x c v i o s

r k j a s d y s d f o l u n k e r j u s d f u w e r t w e m x g p q w i u y s d

j n k u y t w e r l k d f u q w e r u x c b h s d f g b z v x c y t w e r u u s

e b f s u y g e w u a o d p e y x o s d i u d s w x p o t h d k b s k o e i t n

v u e r b n l d k f y u l s k d u s h s e t u t u s k y i u d t h k s d u l o h g

TOTAL Y'S AND I'S _____

ATTENTION

AGING WORDS 3

The answer to each clue contains the letters "AGE."

1. To be enthusiastic and excited about doing something

   ANSWER _____

2. A long journey by sea or through space

   ANSWER _____

3. The remains after destruction

   ANSWER _____

4. Payment for work

   ANSWER _____

5. A measurement used often in football

   ANSWER _____

6. To involve someone in an activity

   ANSWER _____

7. A communication in speech, writing, or signals

   ANSWER _____

8. Used for carrying personal items during a trip

   ANSWER _____

DOMINO ORDER 3

Starting with the domino marked "1st," find an order in which you can line up all these dominoes end to end. Wherever two dominoes touch, the numbered ends must match. You may rotate the dominoes, and there is more than one correct order.

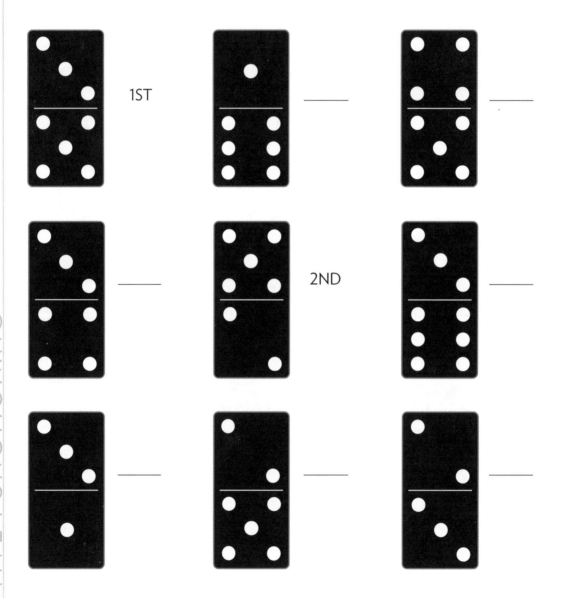

VENN DIAGRAM – MUSIC

Answer the questions using the information displayed in the Venn diagram.

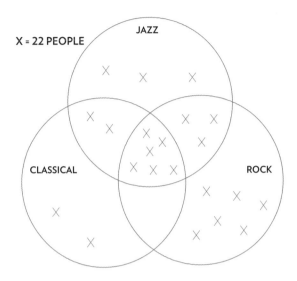

1. How many people like Jazz?

   ANSWER _____

2. How many people like only Jazz?

   ANSWER _____

3. How many people like both Classical and Rock?

   ANSWER _____

4. Which type of music do the most people like?

   ANSWER _____

5. How many people like all three types of music?

   ANSWER _____

6. How many people do not like Rock?

   ANSWER _____

CALENDAR QUIZ 2

Use the calendar clues to determine the correct date.

SUNDAY	MONDAY	TUESDAY	WEDNESDAY	THURSDAY	FRIDAY	SATURDAY
				1	2	3
4	5	6	7	8	9	10
11	12	13	14	15	16	17
18	19	20	21	22	23	24
25	26	27	28	29	30	

1. This date is on a day that begins with "T."

   It is in the last half of the week.

   It is a single-digit date but not 1.

   What is the date? _____

2. This date is not on a weekend.

   It's digits add up to 9.

   It is not Friday the 9th.

   What is the date? _____

EXECUTIVE FUNCTIONING

3. This date is between the 12th and the 21st.

It does not fall on a Monday or Friday.

It is on a Thursday.

What is the date? _____

4. This date is not a double digit.

It is in the middle of the week.

What is the date? _____

DISCOVER THE PATTERN 1

Determine the number sequence pattern and complete the succeeding numbers. You may use a calculator for this excercise

1. 1, 4, 5, 9, 14, 23, _____, _____, _____, _____.

2. 5, 8, 12, 17, 23, _____, _____, _____, _____.

3. 60, 58, 54, 48, 40, _____, _____, _____.

4. 8, 10, 20, 32, 54, _____, _____, _____, _____, _____.

5. 14, 56, 224, 896, _____, _____, _____, _____.

6. 5, 15, 30, 90, 180 _____, _____, _____, _____.

7. 12, 14, 10, 12, 8, _____, _____, _____, _____, _____.

8. 40, 38, 35, 31, _____, _____, _____, _____.

9. 10, 16, 22, 28, _____, _____, _____, _____, _____, _____.

10. 2, 7, 35, 40, 200, _____, _____, _____, _____, _____.

CLOCK QUIZ 1

Use the clues to determine the correct time and then draw it in the clock.

1. This time is in the p.m.

    It is 50 minutes past 2:10.

    What is the time? _____

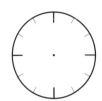

    Draw the clock and the time

2. This time is after noon.

    It is 200 minutes before midnight.

    What is the time? _____

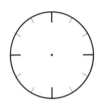

    Draw the clock and the time

3. This time is in the morning.

    It is 915 minutes past noon.

    What is the time? _____

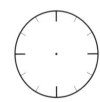

    Draw the clock and the time

4. This time is between 9:30 p.m. and 2:30 a.m.

    It is 345 minutes before 5:00.

    What is the time?_____

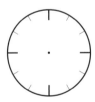

    Draw the clock and the time

TWO COMMON LETTERS 1

Scan each line to find the two letters each word has in common. The letters are next to each other. Challenge yourself to go as quickly as you can.

Example: bounce and balance both have "ce"

COMMON LETTERS

1. jigsaw   jicama   fajita   jinxed   jiggling   _____

2. abrupt   baptize   capture   disrupt   eruption   _____

3. academia empty   condemn   memoir   ceremony   _____

4. eighteen   mightier   tougher   upright   weighted   _____

5. repulse   octopus   punched   tempura   sputter   _____

6. cashew   farewell   firework   renewal   withdrew   _____

7. absolve   involve   twelve   velvet   revolving   _____

8. abiding   edible   hardily   ordinal   dialog   _____

9. corkage   skaters   polka   kashmir   alkaline   _____

10. arranged   barrier   corridor   erratic   marriage   _____

HOW MANY WORDS? 1

How many words can you make out of the letters in the two words below? You can rearrange the letters in any order you want and you do not have to use every letter in each new word.

1. Idiosyncratic

_____

_____

_____

_____

_____

_____

_____

_____

_____

_____

2. Scramble

_____

_____

_____

_____

_____

_____

_____

_____

_____

_____

LANGUAGE

ALLITERATION – CELEBRITIES

Alliteration is when all the words start with the same sound. Complete these sentences with words that begin with the same letter. You can add articles (such as *a*, *an*, *the*) or prepositions (such as *with*, *on*, *as*) to help the sentence make sense.

For example: <u>Mickey Mouse makes me melt.</u>

1. Ronald Reagan _____.

2. Marilyn Monroe _____.

3. _____ muse with Mickey Mantle.

4. _____ joke with Jesse Jackson.

5. Lois Lane _____.

6. _____ swaps Sammy Sosa.

7. LA Lakers _____.

8. Alan Alda _____.

9. _____ beg Bob Barker.

10. Barry Bonds _____.

11. _____ chose Charlie Chaplin.

12. Doris Day _____.

13. Sylvester Stallone _____.

14. Tina Turner _____.

15. _____ hugged Harry Houdini.

LANGUAGE

TWO DEFINITIONS 2

Two definitions for the same word are given. Fill in the correct word that matches both definitions.

1. Not common

   Undercooked

   ANSWER _____

2. A kind of dot

   A Polish dance

   ANSWER _____

3. A stove

   Mountains in a line

   ANSWER _____

4. Finished

   On the other side

   ANSWER _____

5. To propel a boat

   Objects arranged in a straight line

   ANSWER _____

6. A tool used to cut wood

   To see in the past tense

   ANSWER _____

7. The land edge of the ocean

   To glide along

   ANSWER _____

8. To move through the air

   Insect

   ANSWER _____

A BID ON WORDS

The answer to each clue contains the letters "BID."

1. To accept or act in accordance with a rule

   ANSWER _____

2. Relating to disturbing and unpleasant subjects

   ANSWER _____

3. To refuse to allow

   ANSWER _____

4. The sexual drive of a human

   ANSWER _____

5. Having an extreme or fanatical support for or belief in something

   ANSWER _____

6. A bid made in response to a previous bid by another person

   ANSWER _____

IMAGES MEMORY 1

First, spend two minutes studying the images. Then turn the page for a quiz.

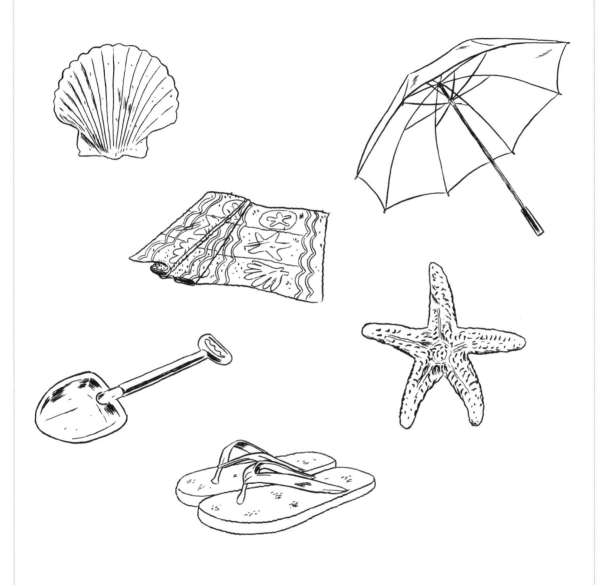

IMAGES MEMORY 1

(DON'T LOOK AT THIS PAGE UNTIL YOU'VE STUDIED PREVIOUS PAGE.)

Now look at the list of words below and circle the words that were images on the previous page.

SHELL

WINDOW

JACKET

TOWEL

UMBRELLA

RAIN

OCEAN

STARFISH

SHARK

SHOVEL

BOOTS

FLIP-FLOPS

FRISBEE

WHAT IS THIS LOCATION?

Determine the location based on the clues.

1. The Florida Air Force base where shuttles are launched

   _____

2. The highest mountain peak on earth _____

3. Disneyland is located in this city _____

4. The birthplace of the cheesesteak _____

5. The home of Mardi Gras _____

6. The Alamo is located here _____

7. The first US national park _____

8. The largest lake in the United States _____

9. The starting point of Route 66 _____

10. Mount Rushmore is carved in the hills of this state

    _____

11. Alcatraz prison sits on an island here _____

12. The USS *Arizona* Memorial is located here in Hawaii

    _____

13. The Hoover Dam is in this state _____

14. The Ellis Island Immigration Museum is here _____

15. This venue in Nashville is known as "the home of American music" and "country music's largest stage"

    _____

MEMORY

COMPLETE THE WORD SEARCH 1

First fill in the answers to the clues, then find those words in the word search grid on the next page. The first letter and number of letters in the word are given.

1. The main ingredient to an omelet   E ____ ____

2. Another word for satire   I ____ ____ ____ ____

3. When something is absolutely necessary
E ____ ____ ____ ____ ____ ____ ____ ____

4. A bar bill is called a   T ____ ____

5. A casino city   R ____ ____ ____

6. When someone is being very open in conversation
C ____ ____ ____ ____ ____

7. Another word for fast   S ____ ____ ____ ____

8. Little girls tie their hair up in a   P ____ ____ ____ ____ ____ ____ ____

9. Part of a suit   V ____ ____ ____

10. You catch butterflies with this   N ____ ____

COMPLETE THE WORD SEARCH 1

Words can be in any direction.

```
A W L B Q R M D J E P R A L
D F Y O V B I C E P M D D Y
G S S K E D N E A E N H G S
W K L P N J I S D S R E W L
A R M A O E U S N A W R A M
H P C I C N L E H O P I H K
R V T C I R Y N Y C O H F T
Q E A L Q E G T P E G G Q T
J S N E T R O I A H K F J N
O T C O F L B A A I R O N Y
M B U N A O P L M T L B M U
B I C B M C K P B A K F B C
G L V V U A V C V B J L G V
```

LETTER-NUMBER SUBSTITUTION CODE 1

Using the code key, determine what words the numbers are spelling.

CODE KEY

A = 16	E = 33	I = 74	M = 67	P = 80	U = 22
C = 24	G = 64	K = 27	N = 42	S = 51	R = 6
D = 44	H = 58	L = 46	O = 92	T = 38	Y = 7

1. 46 16 42 44 67 16 6 27   WORD: _____

2. 24 16 67 16 6 16 44 33 6 74 33   WORD: _____

3. 67 16 6 74 92 42 33 38 38 33   WORD: _____

4. 92 22 38 51 67 16 6 38   WORD: _____

5. 67 16 6 16 38 58 92 42   WORD: _____

6. 44 33 67 16 6 24 16 38 33   WORD: _____

7. 24 22 51 38 92 67 16 6 7   WORD: _____

8. 67 16 6 64 74 42 16 46   WORD: _____

9. 64 6 16 67 67 16 6   WORD: _____

10. 80 6 33 67 16 6 74 38 16 46   WORD: _____

EXECUTIVE FUNCTIONING

MISSPELLED WORDS 1

Pick out the words that are misspelled words, and correct their spelling.

wiegh	_____	adress	_____
calandar	_____	hierarchy	_____
amateur	_____	noticable	_____
libary	_____	balanse	_____
colunm	_____	precede	_____
inoculate	_____	untill	_____
concheince	_____	wheather	_____
cemetery	_____	arguement	_____
excede	_____	beleive	_____
foriegn	_____	indispensable	_____
dicsipline	_____	kernel	_____
miniature	_____	determine	_____
inteligance	_____	leopard	_____

LOGIC WORD PROBLEMS 2

These word problems require you to use the process of elimination to find the answer. It helps to use the grid below.

X = No, not the correct answer; O = Yes, the correct answer

Using the clues, fill in the grid with X's and O's. When there is only one choice left in a row or column, put an O there. Because it is the only option left, it is the correct answer. If a clue tells you the correct choice, you can put an O in that box and put X's in the rest of the column and row because the other options cannot be correct too. Work through all of the clues this way.

1. At a neighbor potluck, there are 5 different kinds of pies. Each friend takes a slice of a different kind of pie. Can you determine which friend chose which pie?

	APPLE	CUSTARD	COCONUT	CHOCOLATE	RASPBERRY
HELEN					
FRANK					
EDDY					
JOYCE					
EMMA					

CLUES
a. Frank is the only one not allergic to coconut.
b. Helen says that chocolate is her therapist.
c. Eddy doesn't like fruit pies.
d. Emma doesn't like getting seeds in her teeth.

2. Some friends are meeting at the park. Each person is taking a different kind of transportation in different colors. Can you determine which person took which type of transportation and in which color?

	CAR	BUS	BIKE	RED	YELLOW	SILVER
LOU						
CONNIE						
STUART						

CLUES
a. Connie loves yellow, but she hates taking public transportation
b. Stuart did not take the red vehicle.
c. Lou had to wear a helmet.

REASONING

WHAT'S THE CATEGORY? 2

Put these words into the most correct category.

baseball   wrench   wire cable   book light
boots   fishing net   a jack   sweatshirts
taillight   helmet   seat cover   adapters
grease   headphones   power cord   umbrella
overalls   camera

1. Things found in the sporting goods section of store

   _____   _____

   _____   _____

   _____   _____

2. Things found in a mechanics repair shop

   _____   _____

   _____   _____

   _____   _____

3. Things found in an electronics store

   _____   _____

   _____   _____

   _____   _____

FIRST AND LAST LETTERS 2

Fill in the correct letters to make a word that matches the definition.

1. ____ isl ____   a church walkway

2. ____ is ____   to stand up

3. ____ as ____   to struggle for breath

4. ____ or ____   additional

5. ____ lad ____   a part of a knife

6. ____ asco ____   a team's symbol

7. ____ es ____   to try it out

8. ____ an ____   a lion's hair

9. ____ di ____   to revise and make changes

10. ____ ti ____   to mix

11. ____ ea ____   letter greeting

12. ____ de ____   you brainstorm this

ORDERED LETTERS 1

Pick the one statement that is WRONG.

1.   ASZCV

A) Z is in the middle.
B) C is after Z.
C) V is at the end.
D) S is between Z and C.

2.   BNDFG

A) N is second.
B) F is between D and G.
C) F is last.
D) D is in the middle.

3.   HJMOK

A) J is to the left of H.
B) M is third.
C) O is between M and K.
D) J is to the right of H.

4.   LPTUI

A) U is between P and I.
B) P is second.
C) L is before P.
D) T is fourth.

5.   QREWY

A) E is right of R.
B) W is left of Y.
C) Q is right of R.
D) Y is last.

6.   UWYVX

A) Y is between W and X.
B) X is not last.
C) V is between Y and X.
D) W is second.

7.   FACNL

A) N is after C.
B) C is left of N.
C) C is right of A.
D) N is between F and C.

8.   JTICD

A) T is before I.
B) C is between T and D.
C) T is left of J.
D) I is in the middle.

SHARED FOOD LETTERS

Write in a letter that completes each word so that a food reads down using your letters.

1. c h a ___ e
  c ___ a s t
  b l ___ e
  ___ a s t

2. a ___ l e
  ___ a t
  l ___ f t
  ___ a l l

3. ___ o m e
  b ___ k e
  k i c ___
  m ___ n u

4. ___ o a p
  b ___ i l
  ___ o u d
  s t ___ r t
  ___ a t e

5. ___ e g u n
  t ___ a i l
  s ___ e d
  r ___ l l y
  b r i ___ e

6. b ___ a i d
  n ___ t u r e
  d r ___ p
  ___ a v e
  p a ___ d
  ___ i c e

7. d i ___ e
  c ___ a t
  d ___ s e
  ___ i t e
  k ___ d
  ___ a s y

8. ___ a ___ h e
  f a ___ m
  d a r ___
  s e ___ l
  s w i ___

9. ___ a i r
  t ___ d e
  v e r ___ e
  ___ a i r

10. n a ___
  t ___ l e
  v ___ s t

LANGUAGE

SHAPE ADDITION

Which shape was added to the first image to create the second image?

1. 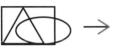 →
   a.   b.   c.   d.

2. →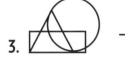
   a.   b.   c.   d.

3. 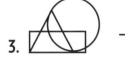 →
   a.   b.   c.   d.

4. 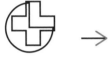 →
   a.   b.   c.   d.

5. →
   a.   b.   c.   d.

6. 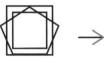 →
   a.   b.   c.   d.

7.  →
   a.   b.   c.   d.

8. →
   a.   b.   c.   d.

PURCHASING PROBLEMS

Determine which items you can buy with the amount you have to spend. Do not worry about including tax. Note: always aim to purchase the most expensive item(s) possible.

1. You have $22.35 to spend on your grandson's birthday present. You want to buy him the most present(s) you can. Choosing the most items possible, which items can you afford to purchase?

BATMAN FIGURE	COLORING BOOK	FOOTBALL	REMOTE CONTROL CAR
$14.79	$3.15	$7.95	$19.05

ANSWER _____

2. You have $70 to spend on new cookware. Choosing the most items possible, which items can you afford to purchase?

SKILLET	CASSEROLE PAN	BOILING POT	SERVING DISH
$30.29	$55.78	$24.35	$14.69

ANSWER _____

3. You have $30 to spend on snacks for the party. Choosing the most items possible, which items can you afford to purchase?

3 OZ. OF CHEESE	4 LBS OF NUTS	2 LBS OF DELI MEAT	12 OZ. OF CRACKERS
AT $5.90 PER OUNCE	AT $3.20 PER POUND	AT $1.25 PER POUND	AT $0.79 PER OUNCE

ANSWER _____

4. You have $7 to spend on office supplies. Choosing the most items possible, which items can you afford to purchase?

10 PENCILS	3 NOTEPADS	CALCULATOR	2 BOXES OF FOLDERS
AT $0.12 EACH	AT $1.15 EACH	$5.65	AT $3.85 EACH

ANSWER _____

CALCULATION

5. You have $25.25 to spend on dinner for four people. Choosing the most items possible, which items can you afford to purchase?

6 LBS OF POTATO	3 LBS OF BEEF	4 LBS OF BROCCOLI	20 OZ. OF RICE
AT $1.32 PER POUND	AT $5.20 PER POUND	AT $0.79 PER POUND	AT $0.32 PER OUNCE

ANSWER _____

6. You have $670 to spend on new furniture. Choosing the most items possible, which items can you afford to purchase?

COUCH	END TABLE	LAMP	ARMCHAIR
$375	$79	$127	$215

ANSWER _____

DECIPHER THE LETTER CODE 4

Complete the phrase by determining the number that is assigned to the used letters.

Begin by filling in the letters that you are given, then figure out which letters make sense to make words in the phrase. You don't have to figure out all the letters, just the ones you need.

For example, if the word is ____ H ____ , the word is likely THE, so 8 = T, therefore you can add in all 8's as T's.
            8   13

A	B	C	D	E	F	G	H	I	J	K	L	M
8		18										15

N	O	P	Q	R	S	T	U	V	W	X	Y	Z
20	14			26	5				22			

MESSAGE:

___ ___ ___ ___   ___ ___ ___   ___ ___ ___ ___ ___ ___
4   8   1   22   8   2   5   22   8   20   24   6   21

___ ___   ___ ___   ___ ___ ___   ___ ___ ___ ___ ___ ,
24   14   13   6   5   14   15   6   13   14   21   2

___ ___ ___   ___ ___ ___   ___   ___ ___ ___ ___ ___ ___ ___
13   11   24   20   14   22   4   26   6   8   1   4   10   6

___   ___ ___ ___ ___ ___ ___   ___ ___ ___ ___   ___ ___ ___ ___
4   5   16   14   11   1   21   16   8   3   6   13   6   6   20

___ ___ ___ ___   ___ ___ ___ ___ ___ ___ ___ ___ .
15   14   26   6   5   7   6   18   4   25   4   18

COUNT THE VOWELS

As quickly as you can, count all of the vowels (a, e, i, o, u) in this paragraph. Scan each line from left to right. Keep a running tally of all letters, don't do one letter at a time.

```
m n d f u s w e r u r y u x g u a d f g u l k j u o i u w e r u s d f u t w e r

j n k u y t w e r l k d f u q w e r u x c b h s d f g b z v x c y t w e r u u s

d f n d l u k s d n f s k d u n k l p u n s d l f y a d f u l j u p i u w e r u p

a u l k d j f i s o d j h u i n d t u t y o e y k f s l y l k j l d f u i n f k s l l

o u w e r u l s u e r u l s i u s l d i u z m c v u z n u d n f u e r y u s d l k

r k j a s d y s d f o l u n k e r j u s d f u w e r t w e m x g p q w i u y s d f

e b f s u y g e w u a o d p e y x o s d i u d s w x p o t h d k b s k o e r t n

f u u n l s u p i u r q w e u l s d f u l k j u l k u k l f s d i f u s d f u x c v

w o q p o w r y r j k u l y s k d n f k s l u k s d n f u k j f k s d n f u n s k

u q w e u u u p o i u q w u a d f u z c v u m b n u k l j h s d f x c v i o s e
```

TOTAL VOWELS _____

AGING WORDS 4

The answer to each clue contains the letters "AGE."

1. A large-scale stage production representing historical events

ANSWER _____

2. To search through things

ANSWER _____

3. To bet on an outcome

ANSWER _____

4. A list of things to do in a specific order

ANSWER _____

5. An actual or mental picture

ANSWER _____

6. A place to keep your car

ANSWER _____

7. A professional representing another person in business

ANSWER _____

8. These fill a book

ANSWER _____

LANGUAGE

DOMINO ORDER 4

Starting with the domino marked "1st," find an order in which you can line up all these domines end to end. Wherever two dominoes touch, the numbered ends must match. You may rotate the dominoes, and there is more than one correct order.

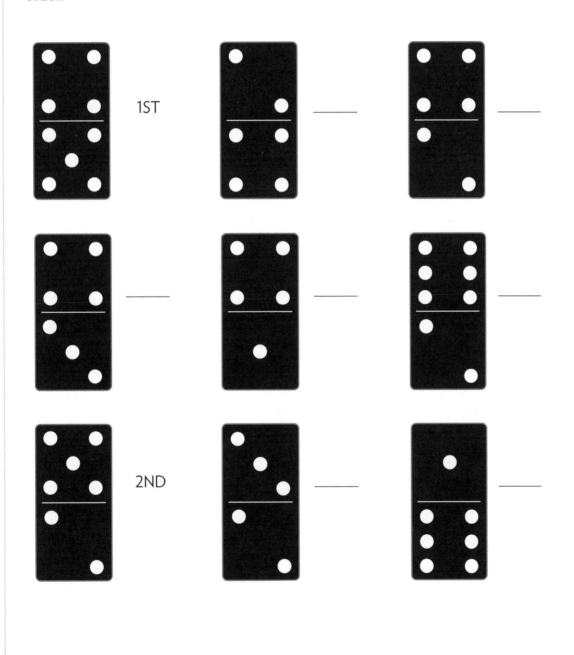

VENN DIAGRAM – TRANSPORTATION

Answer the questions using the information displayed in the Venn diagram.

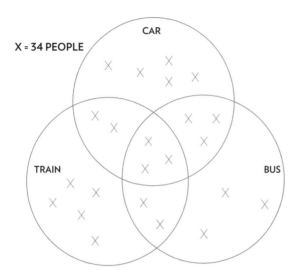

X = 34 PEOPLE

CAR

TRAIN

BUS

1. How many people take the train?

   ANSWER _____

2. Is it more common for people to take the bus or train?

   ANSWER _____

3. How many people take both the bus and drive their car?

   ANSWER _____

4. How many people only drive their car?

   ANSWER _____

5. How many people only take the bus?

   ANSWER _____

6. How many people take all three types of transportation?

   ANSWER _____

VISUAL–SPATIAL

NAME SOMETHING 1

1. Name five professions that start with "P."

_____

_____

_____

_____

_____

2. Name five professions that start with "S."

_____

_____

_____

_____

_____

3. Name five book or movie titles that begin with "M."

_____

_____

_____

_____

_____

LETTERS-TO-WORD MATCH 3

There are 10 six-letter words that have been broken into chunks of three letters. These chunks have been mixed up, no chunk is used twice, and all chunks are used.

Can you determine what the 10 words are?

abs	any	inj	net
dle	hor	bot	lon
mob	joc	kin	urd
ure	don	key	gra
vel	ger	ile	par

1. _____

2. _____

3. _____

4. _____

5. _____

6. _____

7. _____

8. _____

9. _____

10. _____

LANGUAGE

WHAT'S NEXT? 1

Determine which shape comes next in the pattern.

1. à ÿ ÿ ý à ÿ ÿ ý à ÿ
   a. ý   b. à   c. ÿ

2. € £ © © ∞ € £ © © ∞
   a. £   b. €   c. ©

3. ± ± ± ≤ μ μ ± ±
   a. ±   b. ≤   c. μ

4. ¥ ß α ¥ ¥ ß α ¥ ¥
   a. α   b. ß   c. ¥

5. π   barsymbol δ ӽ π barsymbol δ ӽ
   a. π   b. barsymbol   c. δ

6. ϑ ϑ ϑ ß ώ ï ϑ ϑ ϑ ß ώ ï ϑ
   a. ß   b. ώ   c. ϑ

7. Ϛ ς ᴎ ӽ Ϛ ς ᴎ ӽ Ϛ
   a. Ϛ   b. ς   c. ᴎ

CALCULATION WORD PROBLEMS 2

1. While gardening, you have a group of friends come by for a visit. There are 3 women and 2 men. You want to give a bouquet of 6 flowers from your garden to each woman, and a basket of 8 apples from your apple tree to each man. How many total items will you be picking from your garden?

   _____

2. Each time one of your grandchildren visits, you measure their height. Last time Sally was 3 feet 10 inches and Billy was 4 feet 5 inches. Today Sally is 4 feet even, and Billy is 4 feet 8 inches. How many total inches did they both grow together?

   _____ inches

3. You are going to bring pies to a neighborhood potluck. There are going to be 28 people attending. If each pie yields 6 slices, how many pies should you bring so that everyone can get at least one piece?

   _____ pies

4. Your family drinks one gallon of milk every 4 days. At the grocery store, you want to buy enough milk to last for at least 2 weeks. How many gallons of milk should you buy?

   _____ gallons

5. You need to buy a large floor carpet for your living room. It needs to be twice as long in length as the width. The width should be 8 feet. How long should the length of the carpet be?

   _____ feet

6. You want to walk 2 ½ miles each day. The distance around your block is ¼ of a mile. How many times would you have to walk around your block in one day to accomplish your goal?

   _____

ACCOMPLISH THIS TASK 1

Determine two different ways you could accomplish each task. There is not one right answer, so be as creative as you like.

Keep papers together
1. _____
2. _____

Hang a picture
1. _____
2. _____

Join two pieces of wood
1. _____
2. _____

Grow a garden
1. _____
2. _____

Build a tent
1. _____
2. _____

Make a quilt
1. _____
2. _____

Give a gift
1. _____
2. _____

Climb a hill
1. _____
2. _____

Travel across country
1. _____
2. _____

Pay for a purchase
1. _____
2. _____

Renew a library book
1. _____
2. _____

REASONING

BAD WORDS

The answer to each clue contains the letters "BAD."

1. A small distinctive piece of metal to show rank

   ANSWER _____

2. To order someone not to do something; not allow (past tense)

   ANSWER _____

3. A game with nets and rackets

   ANSWER _____

4. A burrowing mammal related to the weasel

   ANSWER _____

5. To criticize or make disparaging remarks about somebody

   ANSWER _____

6. A medieval poet or singer of lyric verses about love, who performs while strolling

   ANSWER _____

MATCH THE PARTS 1

Match a word-part on the left with a word-part on the right to form a word and write it on the line. You can only use each word-part once.

1. dan   any   _____

     acc   mal   _____

     lea   ade   _____

     for   cer   _____

     bot   son   _____

     par   use   _____

     can   der   _____

     rea   ary   _____

2. enl   gie   _____

     cav   ium   _____

     hoa   ear   _____

     inv   ive   _____

     lin   ist   _____

     sod   ity   _____

     act   lic   _____

     fro   ent   _____

TWO COMMON LETTERS 2

Scan each line to find the two letters each word has in common. The letters are next to each other. Challenge yourself to go as quickly as you can.

Example: bounce and balance both have "ce"

COMMON LETTERS

1.	faith	infant	loofah	safari	unfair	_____
2.	amoeba	nebula	debtor	rebate	zebra	_____
3.	brain	afraid	cobra	brandy	corals	_____
4.	amount	county	fungus	hunter	ounce	_____
5.	eject	deduct	action	victim	sector	_____
6.	compass	impair	keypad	pajama	unpaid	_____
7.	muscle	escrow	rescue	scents	rascal	_____
8.	thirdly	stirrup	upstairs	twirled	wiring	_____
9.	barley	eyelids	survey	hockey	obeying	_____
10.	hourly	pearl	burlap	uncurl	worldly	_____

DISCOVER THE PATTERN 2

Determine the number sequence pattern and complete the succeeding numbers. You may use a calculator for this excercise.

1. 2, 6, 10, ———, ———, ———, ———.

2. 5, 10, 20, 40, ———, ———, ———, ———.

3. 3, 5, 4, 6, ———, ———, ———, ———, ———.

4. 8, 12, 10, 14, 12, ———, ———, ———, ———, ———.

5. 8, 32, 16, 64, ———, ———, ———, ———, ———.

6. 3, 9, 6, 18, 15, ———, ———, ———, ———, ———.

7. 5, 10, 10, 15, 15, ———, ———, ———, ———, ———.

8. 12, 14, 15, 18, 17, 21, ———, ———, ———, ———, ———.

9. 4, 8, 4, 12, 4, 16, ———, ———, ———, ———, ———, ———.

10. 6, 6, 12, 36, ———, ———, ———, ———.

COMPOUND WORDS 1

Make as many compound words as you can with these beginnings.

1. be _____

   be _____

   be _____

   be _____

   be _____

   be _____

   be _____

   be _____

2. in _____

   in _____

   in _____

   in _____

   in _____

   in _____

   in _____

   in _____

3. out _____

   out _____

   out _____

   out _____

   out _____

   out _____

   out _____

   out _____

   out _____

   out _____

   out _____

   out _____

   out _____

   out _____

MEMORY

SYMBOL CODING 3

Write the symbol that corresponds to each number in the empty boxes below. Challenge yourself to do this as quickly as you can, while maintaining accuracy. Do not do all of one number at a time, complete each box in a row moving from left to right, and then continue to the next line.

KEY CODE

1	2	3	4	5	6	7	8	9
□	×	⊔	◇	△	↑	—	○	+

7	9	3	1	4	2	7	8	5	6
4	1	6	8	2	9	3	5	4	2
5	9	1	4	2	7	5	9	8	6
3	6	7	8	3	4	9	1	2	5
7	9	3	1	4	2	7	8	5	6
6	3	1	7	2	5	9	8	2	1
2	9	8	5	1	4	7	3	6	8
1	5	7	4	3	6	2	1	9	3

SEQUENCING ITEMS 2

Discover a logical way to sequence these items, and explain the *reason* why you put them in that order. No alphabetical order allowed.

1. Rough draft, Outline, Final copy, Editing

   1st _____ 2nd _____ 3rd _____ 4th _____

   Reason _____

2. Precipitation, Condensation, Evaporation, Accumulation

   1st _____ 2nd _____ 3rd _____ 4th _____

   Reason _____

3. Bird, Plankton, Fish, Cat

   1st _____ 2nd _____ 3rd _____ 4th _____

   Reason _____

4. Novel, Flyer, Pamphlet, Paragraph

   1st _____ 2nd _____ 3rd _____ 4th _____

   Reason _____

5. Basement, Roof, Attic, Foundation

   1st _____ 2nd _____ 3rd _____ 4th _____

   Reason _____

6. Ford, Kennedy, Bush, Reagan

   1st _____ 2nd _____ 3rd _____ 4th _____

   Reason _____

7. Texas, Rhode Island, Ohio, Vermont

   1st _____ 2nd _____ 3rd _____ 4th _____

   Reason _____

8. Election, Ballot counting, Nomination, Voting

1st _____ 2nd _____ 3rd _____ 4th _____

Reason _____

9. Ankle, Forehead, Waist, Thigh

1st _____ 2nd _____ 3rd _____ 4th _____

Reason _____

10. Take home, Customer, Store, Purchase

1st _____ 2nd _____ 3rd _____ 4th _____

Reason _____

11. Blueberry, Avocado, Cantaloupe, Mushroom

1st _____ 2nd _____ 3rd _____ 4th _____

Reason _____

12. Rosa Parks, *Apollo 11*, Nixon resigns, The Beatles come to America

1st _____ 2nd _____ 3rd _____ 4th _____

Reason _____

13. Appeal, Hearing, Sentencing, Trial

1st _____ 2nd _____ 3rd _____ 4th _____

Reason _____

14. Atom, Element, Electron, Molecule

1st _____ 2nd _____ 3rd _____ 4th _____

Reason _____

WORDS THAT CAN

The answer to each clue contains the letters "CAN."

1. Empty; having no furniture or inhabitants

   ANSWER _____

2. An action or event regarded as morally or legally wrong and causing general public outrage

   ANSWER _____

3. A narrow boat with pointed ends, propelled by paddles

   ANSWER _____

4. Truthful; straightforward; frank

   ANSWER _____

5. A brown nut with an edible kernel

   ANSWER _____

6. A cylinder block of wax with a wick

   ANSWER _____

7. To decide or announce that an event will not take place

   ANSWER _____

8. A strong coarse cloth used for sails, tents, or paintings

   ANSWER _____

LANGUAGE

FAMILY TREE GAME 2

Based on this family tree, answer the questions below with a specific name.

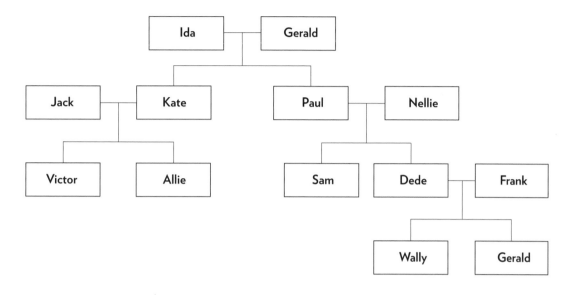

1. Who is Dede's grandmother? _____

2. Who is Kate's sister-in-law? _____

3. Who is the youngest Gerald named after? _____

4. Who are Ida's grandsons? _____

5. Who is Paul's sister's daughter? _____

6. Who is Wally's grandfather? _____

MATCHING CLUES 3

Match two of the word-parts to make a word that fits the clue. Each word-part is used only once.

loc   ck   ak   nap

kin   mo   ket   pe

1. _____ a small ornamental case

_____ to tease

_____ a square piece of cloth

_____ greatest; maximun

ken   ket   ta   nk

pac   sil   pra   sk

2. _____ a container

_____ duty

_____ a mischievous joke

_____ soft and lustrous

LANGUAGE

WHAT'S THE CATEGORY? 3

Put these words into the most correct category.

zippers	tubes	checks	tellers
slides	hangers	vault	mothballs
hooks	change	photo albums	goggles
eyewash kit	loans	element chart	funnels
hat box	interest		

1. Things found in a closet

2. Things found in a science lab

3. Things found in a bank

ORDERED LETTERS 2

Pick the one statement that is CORRECT.

1. **ASZCV**

    A) C is fifth.
    B) C is between A and Z.
    C) S is between A and Z.
    D) V is not last.

2. **BNDFG**

    A) D is right of F.
    B) F is left of G.
    C) F is last.
    D) D is first.

3. **HJMOK**

    A) O is between H and M.
    B) M is not in the middle.
    C) K is left of O.
    D) J is right of H.

4. **LPTUI**

    A) U is between T and L.
    B) P is left of L.
    C) L is left of P.
    D) T is fourth.

5. **QREWY**

    A) W is left of Y.
    B) R is left of Q.
    C) R is left of Q.
    D) E is fourth.

6. **UWYVX**

    A) V is right of X.
    B) W is right of V.
    C) V is between U and Y.
    D) Y is right of W.

7. **FACNL**

    A) C is after N.
    B) A is left of C.
    C) C is right of A.
    D) N is between F and C.

8. **JTICD**

    A) J is right of C.
    B) I is between J and C.
    C) T is left of J.
    D) D is left of C.

EXECUTIVE FUNCTIONING

WHAT'S THE ITEM? 2

Determine what item these clues are describing and write it on the line.

1. This stuff lies all around our houses.

   We don't like to see it around, so we wipe it up.

   Scientists say it is mostly made of dead skin cells.

   What is this item? ⎯⎯⎯⎯⎯⎯⎯⎯⎯⎯⎯⎯⎯⎯⎯

2. Today kids like to use these for crafts.

   Their original purpose was to dry clothes.

   You use them on a line outside.

   What are these items? ⎯⎯⎯⎯⎯⎯⎯⎯⎯⎯⎯⎯⎯⎯⎯

3. You can use this to drink.

   It usually comes in a glass.

   Some people like to chew on them.

   What is this item? ⎯⎯⎯⎯⎯⎯⎯⎯⎯⎯⎯⎯⎯⎯⎯

4. These are small and round.

   They are made to fit through holes.

   They can keep your shirt on.

   What are these items? ⎯⎯⎯⎯⎯⎯⎯⎯⎯⎯⎯⎯⎯⎯⎯

5. These are made of porous material.

   They are used to clean up liquid.

   They can be squeezed out.

   What are these items? ⎯⎯⎯⎯⎯⎯⎯⎯⎯⎯⎯⎯⎯⎯⎯

REASONING

CLOCK QUIZ 2

Use the clues to determine the correct time and then draw it in the clock.

1. This time is not in the a.m.

   It is 98 minutes past 2:00.

   What is the time? _____

Draw the clock and the time

2. This time is before lunch.

   It falls between 6:00 and 8:00.

   It is 390 minutes past midnight.

   What is the time? _____

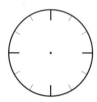

Draw the clock and the time

3. This time is at night.

   It 560 minutes past noon.

   What is the time? _____

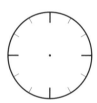

Draw the clock and the time

4. This time is between 2:30 a.m. and 2:30 p.m.

   It is 45 minutes before 6:15.

   What is the time? _____

Draw the clock and the time

EXECUTIVE FUNCTIONING

DECIPHER THE LETTER CODE 5

Complete the phrase by determining the number that is assigned to the used letters.

Begin by filling in the letters that you are given, then figure out which letters make sense to make words in the phrase. You don't have to figure out all the letters, just the ones you need.

For example, if the word is ____ H ____ , the word is likely THE, so 8 = T,
                           8   13

therefore you can add in all 8's as T's.

A	B	C	D	E	F	G	H	I	J	K	L	M
	13	17		3						6		16

N	O	P	Q	R	S	T	U	V	W	X	Y	Z
	23	4			10					11		

MESSAGE:

____ ____ ____ ____ ____ ____ ____ ____ ____   ____ ____ ____ ____
 5   17 23 16   4   2   25   3   24   23 14 17   3

____ ____ ____ ____   ____ ____   ____ ____   ____ ____ ____ ____ ____ ,
 13   3   5   25   16   3   5   25   17   1   3   10   10

____ ____ ____   ____ ____   ____ ____ ____   ____ ____
 13   2   25   20   25   21   5   10   14   23

____ ____ ____ ____ ____   ____ ____ ____   ____ ____   ____ ____
 16   5   25   17   1   9   23   24   16   3   5   25

____ ____ ____ ____ ____ ____ ____ ____ ____ .
 6   20   17   6   13   23   11   20   14   19

COUNT THE CONSONANTS

As quickly as you can, count all of the consonants (any letter that is not a vowel) in this paragraph. Scan each line from left to right. Keep a running tally of all letters, don't do one letter at a time.

a e i f u s w e r u r y u x g u a d f a e o k j u o i u w e r u s d f u t w e r

j a k u y t w e r l a e o u q w e r u x c b a e l f g a z v x c a t w e r u u s

d f a e l u k s d n f s k d u a e l p u n s a l f y a d f u l j u p i u w e r u p

a u l k a j f i s o a a h u i n d t u t y o e y a f s a y l k a l a f u i n f k s a l

o u w e r u a s u e r u a s i u e o d i u z m c v u z n u d n f u e r y u s d l

r k j a s d y s e d f o l u n k e r j u s e f u w e r t w e m x g p q w i u y s

e b o s u y g e w u a o d p e y x o s d i u d s w x p o t h e k a s k o e r t n

f u u n l s u p i u r q w e u l s d f u l k j u l k u k l f s d i f u s d f u x c v

w o q e o w r y r j k u l y s k d n f a s l u k s d n f u a j e k s d n e u n s k

u q w e u a u p o i u q w u a d f u z c v u m e i u k l j h s d f x c v i o s e

TOTAL CONSONANTS _____

ATTENTION

WORDS FULL OF AWE

The answer to each clue contains the letters "AWE."

1. You do this to a domesticated house pet to prevent damage to your furniture

   ANSWER _____

2. To be filled with overwhelming emotion; enthralled, captivated

   ANSWER _____

3. A storage compartment in a piece of furniture

   ANSWER _____

4. Having imperfections

   ANSWER _____

5. To chew at something persistently (past tense)

   ANSWER _____

6. To make illegal (past tense)

   ANSWER _____

7. Plants that grow in the ocean

   ANSWER _____

8. To melt something (past tense)

   ANSWER _____

DOT COPY 2

Copy these patterns onto the blank graphs.

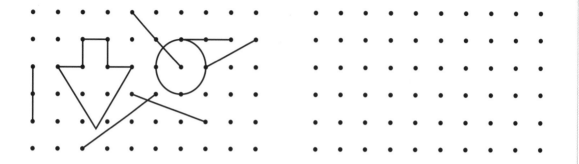

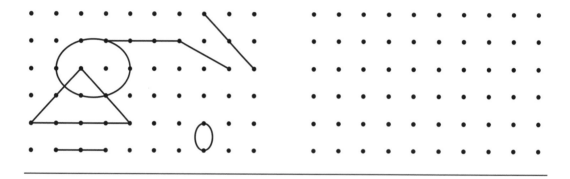

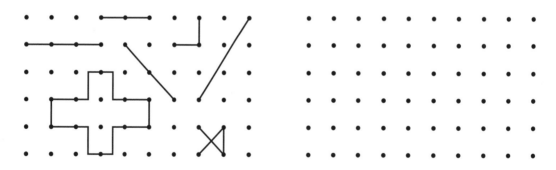

VISUAL–SPATIAL

NAME SOMETHING 2

1. Name five countries that start with "C."

   _____

   _____

   _____

   _____

   _____

2. Name five drinks that start with "G."

   _____

   _____

   _____

   _____

   _____

3. Name five things that begin with "Y."

   _____

   _____

   _____

   _____

   _____

LOGIC WORD PROBLEMS 3

These word problems require you to use the process of elimination to find the answer. It helps to use the grid below.

X = No, not the correct answer; O = Yes, the correct answer

Using the clues, fill in the grid with X's and O's. When there is only one choice left in a row or column, put an O there. Because it is the only option left, it is the correct answer. If a clue tells you the correct choice, you can put an O in that box and put X's in the rest of the column and row because the other options cannot be correct too. Work through all of the clues this way.

1. Five people are waiting in line at the grocery store. What is the order of the line?

	FIRST	SECOND	THIRD	FOURTH	FIFTH
SARAH					
WALTER					
ABBY					
NEAL					
MALLORY					

CLUES
a. Abby is not first or last.
b. Abby is directly in front of Mallory.
c. Walter is in the middle.
d. Sarah is after Neal.

2. Lori, Amy, Hank, and Randy went out dancing together. Each danced a different type of dance with a partner not in their group. Can you determine who danced which type of dance and with whom?

	LEO	JANE	BRIAN	NATALIE	JITTERBUG	SALSA	SWING	LINDY HOP
LORI								
AMY								
HANK								
RANDY								

CLUES

a. Each person danced with a partner of the opposite sex.

b. Hank did not do the jitterbug nor dance with Natalie.

c. Lori danced with a man who has the same letter as her name to a dance with the same letter as her name.

d. Randy loves to salsa dance.

TWO DEFINITIONS 3

Two definitions for the same word are given. Fill in the correct word that matches both definitions.

1. He goes out of a place; he . . .

   They grow on trees

   ANSWER _____

2. Remaining

   Not right

   ANSWER _____

3. A hammer hits it

   It grows on your finger

   ANSWER _____

4. To not eat for a determined time

   Quick

   ANSWER _____

5. To put in alphabetical order

   It smooths out an edge

   ANSWER _____

6. A formal dance

   A round object

   ANSWER _____

7. A measure of weight

   A home for lost dogs

   ANSWER _____

8. To be unkind

   Average

   ANSWER _____

LANGUAGE

EDIT THE WORD 1

In the first column, change one letter in the original word to make a new word. In the second column, take out one letter from the original word and keep the rest of the letters in the same order to form a new word.

For example:

	CHANGE ONE LETTER	TAKE OUT ONE LETTER
Spank	Spark	Sank

		CHANGE ONE LETTER	TAKE OUT ONE LETTER
1.	Table	_____	_____
2.	Hurt	_____	_____
3.	Race	_____	_____
4.	Tail	_____	_____
5.	Fuse	_____	_____
6.	Scan	_____	_____
7.	Bark	_____	_____
8.	Tank	_____	_____

LANGUAGE

ACCOMPLISH THIS TASK 2

Determine two things you would need to accomplish each task. There is not one right answer, so be as creative as you like.

For example: To fill a prescription, you would need

1. A physician's signature, and 2. patience for the line at the pharmacy.

Dial a phone
1. _____
2. _____

Make coffee
1. _____
2. _____

Grocery shop
1. _____
2. _____

Wrap a gift
1. _____
2. _____

Go on a date
1. _____
2. _____

Take a photo
1. _____
2. _____

Play a game
1. _____
2. _____

Feed your pet
1. _____
2. _____

Take a nap
1. _____
2. _____

Play an instrument
1. _____
2. _____

REASONING

Use a flashlight   1. _____

2. _____

Write a check   1. _____

2. _____

Wash your hair   1. _____

2. _____

Keep a secret   1. _____

2. _____

Ride a bike   1. _____

2. _____

Hem a dress   1. _____

2. _____

Go swimming   1. _____

2. _____

Bake a cake   1. _____

2. _____

Put out a fire   1. _____

2. _____

Replace a lightbulb   1. _____

2. _____

Make ice   1. _____

2. _____

Walk around the block   1. _____

2. _____

Tell a joke   1. _____

2. _____

LETTER TRANSFER 3

Fill in the word to answer the clue, then transfer those numbered letters to the lines on the next page for the final message.

1. What the "F" stands for in FBI

    ___ ___ ___ ___ ___ ___ ___
     1   2   3   2   4   5   6

2. Tony Curtis was in this armed service during World War II

    ___ ___ ___ ___
     7   5   8   9

3. In the charity AHA, what body part does the 'H' stand for

    ___ ___ ___ ___ ___
    12   2   5   4 13

4. Kennedy and Johnson both died in this state

    ___ ___ ___ ___ ___
    13   2 14   5 15

5. This state is called the Golden State

    ___ ___ ___ ___ ___ ___ ___ ___ ___ ___
    16   5   6 17   1 18   4   7 17   5

MEMORY

6. This state is called the Aloha State

———— ———— ———— ———— ———— ————
12   5   19   5   17   17

7. The past tense of the word "swing"

———— ———— ———— ———— ————
15   19   20   7   21

FINAL MESSAGE:

———— ———— ————   ———— ———— ———— ————   ———— ————   ———— ———— ———— ———— ———— ———— ————
13 12 2   4 18 5 3   13 18   15 20 16 16 2 15 15

———— ————   ———— ———— ———— ———— ———— ————   ———— ———— ———— ———— ————
17 15   5 6 19 5 9 15   20 7 3 2 4

———— ———— ———— ———— ———— ———— ———— ———— ———— ———— ———— ———— .
16 18 7 15 13 4 20 16 13 17 18 7

A CUP OF WORDS

The answer to each clue contains the letters "CUP."

1. A job or profession

ANSWER _____

2. To recover from illness or exertion

ANSWER _____

3. A cabinet with shelves for storage

ANSWER _____

4. A classical mythological character known as the son of the goddess of love

ANSWER _____

5. An involuntary spasm of the diaphragm making a sudden sound

ANSWER _____

6. To reside in a location

ANSWER _____

7. A large rodent with defensive quills on its body

ANSWER _____

CODING – OCCUPATIONS

Use the key code below to decode the words. Each space is one letter. Challenge yourself to go as quickly as you can. All of these words are in the category: **OCCUPATIONS**.

1. PHYSICIAN

2. TEACHER

3. ACCOUNTANT

4. ELECTRICIAN

5. PILOT

KEY CODE

A	B	C	D	E	F	G	H	I	J	K	L	M

N	O	P	Q	R	S	T	U	V	W	X	Y	Z

LOGIC WORD PROBLEMS 4

These word problems require you to use the process of elimination to find the answer. It helps to use the grid below.

X = No, not the correct answer; O = Yes, the correct answer

Using the clues, fill in the grid with X's and O's. When there is only one choice left in a row or column, put an O there. Because it is the only option left, it is the correct answer. If a clue tells you the correct choice, you can put an O in that box and put X's in the rest of the column and row because the other options cannot be correct too. Work through all of the clues this way.

1. Sally, Rick, Jay, and Beverly were playing a card game. They had to figure out which person had the ace of spades, jack of hearts, queen of clubs, and king of diamonds. Can you determine which person had which card?

	ACE/SPADES	JACK/HEARTS	QUEEN/CLUBS	KING/DIAMONDS
SALLY				
RICK				
JAY				
BEVERLY				

CLUES

a. Jay did not have a heart or club.

b. Rick was the only person to have a spade.

c. Sally wished she had a queen because they were always her lucky cards.

REASONING

2. Five friends were shopping for home goods together. Which person bought which item at the store?

	LAWN CHAIR	HAMMER	SCISSORS	DOOR HINGE	WRENCH
HARRY					
EMMA					
JOANNE					
LEO					
DIANE					

CLUES
a. Joanne had already replaced all her old creaky door hinges last month and didn't need any now, but she had some good advice for Leo.

b. Emma was in the middle of a sewing project when she realized she needed a supply.

c. Harry did not need any tools, but Joanne did.

d. Diane needed a different size wrench for her project.

ORDERED NUMBERS 1

Pick the one statement that is WRONG.

1. 53691

A) 3 is second.
B) 9 is between 6 and 1.
C) 5 is not first.
D) 6 is in the middle.

2. 74182

A) 4 is after 1.
B) 1 is in the middle.
C) 8 is between 4 and 2.
D) 8 is fourth.

3. 64823

A) 8 Is right of 4.
B) 2 is left of 3.
C) 4 is between 6 and 3.
D) 3 is fourth.

4. 91734

A) 3 is between 4 and 7.
B) 7 is fourth.
C) 9 is before 1.
D) 3 is right of 7.

5. 67928

A) 2 is right of 6.
B) 6 is left of 2.
C) 9 is in the middle.
D) 8 is not last.

6. 35421

A) 2 is between 1 and 4.
B) 4 is left of 2.
C) 1 is right of 2.
D) 2 is fifth.

7. 65283

A) 2 is after 8.
B) 5 is left of 2.
C) 8 is right of 5.
D) 8 is fourth.

8. 57139

A) 7 is between 3 and 5.
B) 3 is right of 1.
C) 1 is right of 9.
D) 1 is in the middle.

EXECUTIVE FUNCTIONING

MATCHING CLUES 4

Match two of the word-parts to make a word that fits the clue. Each word-part is used only once.

rk   shi   thi   spa

ver   tch   ske   nk

1. _____ a rough drawing

   _____ to shake slightly

   _____ a small fiery particle

   _____ to ponder

yo   ck   ke   sli

nk   wic   ya   ker

2. _____ smooth and glossy

   _____ to pull with a jerk

   _____ woven twigs

   _____ a wooden crosspiece

START HERE – END THERE

Find at least three ways to get from the first number to the second number. You may use any combination of operations: addition (+), subtraction (-), multiplication (x), or division (/) to reach your goal. Remember the order of operations when working out an equation: First do any multiplication and division (working left to right), then do any addition and subtraction (working left to right).

For example: 8   = 27

$$8 + 20 - 1 = 27 \qquad 8 \times 3 + 3 = 27 \qquad 8 / 2 + 23 = 27$$

This column must include:

	ADDITION & SUBTRACTION	MULTIPLICATION	DIVISION
1. 2 = 15			
2. 3 = 17			
3. 4 = 22			
4. 5 = 48			
5. 6 = 74			
6. 7 = 88			
7. 8 = 30			
8. 9 = 25			
9. 10 = 48			

CALCULATION

Now you can use any combination of operations you choose:

10. 12 = 62 _____ _____ _____

11. 15 = 86 _____ _____ _____

12. 24 = 92 _____ _____ _____

WORDS THAT FIT

The answer to each clue contains the letters "FIT."

1. To receive an advantage; gain

   ANSWER _____

2. A person whose behavior or attitude sets them apart from others in an uncomfortably conspicuous way

   ANSWER _____

3. A set of clothing worn together for a particular occasion

   ANSWER _____

4. A financial gain or advantage

   ANSWER _____

5. To add a component to a product that did not have it when manufactured

   ANSWER _____

6. A writing or drawing sprayed illicitly on a wall in a public place

   ANSWER _____

7. To be appropriate for

   ANSWER _____

8. The condition of being physically healthy

   ANSWER _____

LETTERS-TO-WORD MATCH 4

There are 10 six-letter words that have been broken into chunks of three letters. These chunks have been mixed up, no chunk is used twice and all chunks are used.

Can you determine what the 10 words are?

cha	orc	cac	ace
tus	att	sec	anc
sce	hid	rge	tic
ach	hor	pal	lau
kle	nch	ret	nic

1. _____

2. _____

3. _____

4. _____

5. _____

6. _____

7. _____

8. _____

9. _____

10. _____

SYMBOL CODING 4

Write the number that corresponds to each symbol in the empty boxes below. Challenge yourself to do this as quickly as you can, while maintaining accuracy. Do not do all of one symbol at a time, complete each box in a row moving from left to write, and then continue to the next line.

KEY CODE

ꜱ	ᴫ	℺	ꜿ	Ξ	Δ	Ⱶ	ᴎ	ꭓ
5	9	3	2	4	7	1	8	6

Δ	ꜿ	Ξ	ꜱ	ᴎ	ᴫ	Ⱶ	ꭓ	℺	ꜱ
Ξ	ᴎ	Ⱶ	ᴫ	Δ	℺	ꭓ	ꜱ	ᴎ	ꜿ
Ⱶ	ꜱ	℺	ꭓ	ꜿ	Ξ	Δ	ᴎ	ᴫ	Ⱶ
ᴫ	Δ	ᴎ	Ⱶ	ꭓ	Δ	ꜱ	ꜿ	℺	Ξ
ꜱ	Ⱶ	ꭓ	P	Ξ	ᴎ	ᴫ	ꭓ	Δ	Ⱶ
ꜿ	ᴎ	ᴫ	ꜱ	Δ	Ⱶ	ꭓ	℺	Ξ	ᴫ
P	ꭓ	Δ	Ⱶ	ᴎ	ꭓ	℺	ꜱ	Ⱶ	Δ

SUNNY WORDS

The answer to each clue contains the letters "SUN."

1. An ice cream dessert with toppings

    ANSWER _____

2. Submerged beneath the surface of the water

    ANSWER _____

3. To lie outside to get a tan

    ANSWER _____

4. Not praised or honored, such as an _____ hero

    ANSWER _____

5. A piece of women's clothing worn in hot weather

    ANSWER _____

6. Protects skin from damaging UV rays

    ANSWER _____

7. A large destructive ocean wave

    ANSWER _____

8. An instrument that shows time by using shadows

    ANSWER _____

CALENDAR QUIZ 3

Use the calendar clues to determine the correct date.

SUNDAY	MONDAY	TUESDAY	WEDNESDAY	THURSDAY	FRIDAY	SATURDAY
	1	2	3	4	5	6
7	8	9	10	11	12	13
14	15	16	17	18	19	20
21	22	23	24	25	26	27
28	29	30	31			

1. This date is on a day that begins with "S."

   It is in the middle week of the month.

   It is not the 20th.

   What is the date? _____

2. This date is not on a weekday.

   It is a single digit.

   It is not on a Sunday.

   What is the date? _____

EXECUTIVE FUNCTIONING

3. This date is between the 21st and the 31st.

It is on a Wednesday.

It is not the last day of the month.

What is the date? _____

4. This date is in the first half of the month.

It is in the middle of the week.

It is not the 3rd.

What is the date? _____

Scan each line to find the two letters each word has in common. The letters are next to each other. Challenge yourself to go as quickly as you can.

Example: bounce and balance both have "ce"

COMMON LETTERS

1. allegory egotist illegal neglect vinegar _____

2. allocate bachelor cloister employee lockable _____

3. caffeine divinity finalist linger ceiling _____

4. crumple entrust grueling protrude ruminate _____

5. leftovers aircraft grifters shoplift softness _____

6. disrobe newsroom misread pressrun misrule _____

7. billiard ambrosia cardiac enviable partial _____

8. ensemble amenable dribble humble blue _____

9. betrayer doctrine atrocity geometry mistrust _____

10. bicycle diabolical efficacy evicted justice _____

PROCESSING SPEED

CLOCK QUIZ 3

Use the clues to determine the correct time and then draw it in the clock.

1. This time is in the p.m.

   It is 80 minutes past 8:25.

   What is the time? _____

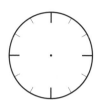

Draw the clock and the time

2. This time is in the morning.

   It is 145 minutes after 1:35.

   What is the time? _____

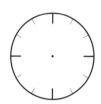

Draw the clock and the time

3. This time is not in the afternoon.

   It is 425 minutes past midnight.

   What is the time? _____

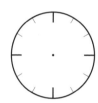

Draw the clock and the time

4. This time is between 1:00 a.m. and 1:00 p.m.

   It is 130 minutes before 3:00.

   What is the time? _____

Draw the clock and the time

HOW MANY WORDS? 2

How many words can you make out of the letters in the two words below? You can rearrange the letters in any order you want and you do not have to use every letter in each new word.

1. Accoutrement

_____

_____

_____

_____

_____

_____

_____

_____

_____

_____

2. Gardening

_____

_____

_____

_____

_____

_____

_____

_____

_____

_____

LANGUAGE

FURRY WORDS

The answer to each clue contains the letters "FUR."

1. A yellow combustible chemical element that smells bad

   ANSWER _____

2. To make or become spread out from a rolled or folded state

   ANSWER _____

3. An appliance fired by gas, oil, or wood in which air or water is heated

   ANSWER _____

4. Extremely angry

   ANSWER _____

5. To renovate and redecorate a building

   ANSWER _____

6. Large movable objects to make a space suitable for living or working

   ANSWER _____

7. A leave of absence granted to a member of the military

   ANSWER _____

MIDDLE LETTERS 2

Fill in the correct letters to make a word that matches the definition.

1. s _____ _____ _____ e   to look happy

2. h _____ n   the source of an egg

3. e _____ _____ o   when a sound reverberates

4. u _____ _____ _____ _____ _____ l   a fork, spoon, or knife

5. d _____ _____ i   a sandwich store

6. e _____ _____ _____ _____ _____ n   a feeling

7. a _____ _____ _____ s   pains

8. s _____ _____ _____ _____ _____ s   spring, summer, fall, winter

9. p _____ _____ h   a garden walkway

10. s _____ _____ _____ _____ _____ e   a soup cracker

11. c _____ _____ t   an informal talk

12. s _____ _____ _____ d   swiftness

MEMORY CROSSWORD 1

First, spend two minutes studying the words in this crossword. Then turn the page for a quiz.

MEMORY CROSSWORD 1

(DON'T LOOK AT THIS PAGE UNTIL YOU'VE STUDIED PREVIOUS PAGE.)

Now look at the list of words below and circle the words that were in the crossword on the previous page.

GLORY

POKER

NEAR

AMUSE

ENTERTAIN

BATTLE

RECEIVE

REPAIR

POSTAGE

SENDER

CASINO

GALLOP

REWARD

IMAGES MEMORY 2

First, spend two minutes studying the images. Then turn the page for a quiz.

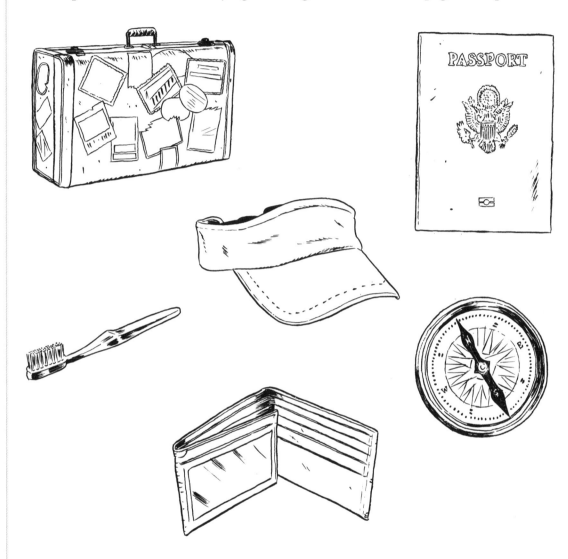

IMAGES MEMORY 2

(DON'T LOOK AT THIS PAGE UNTIL YOU'VE STUDIED PREVIOUS PAGE.)

Now look at the list of words below and circle the words that were images on the previous page.

VISOR

COMPUTER

TICKET

PASSPORT

AIRPLANE

UMBRELLA

SUITCASE

TOOTHBRUSH

MAP

COMPASS

SHOES

JOURNAL

WALLET

DOT COPY 3

Copy these patterns onto the blank graphs.

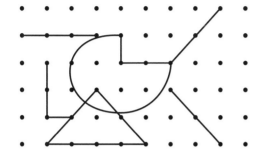

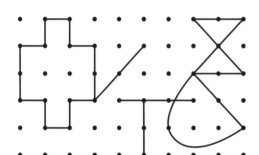

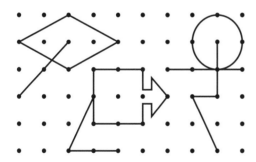

VISUAL-SPATIAL

"D" WORDS

Using two clues, fill in the correct word that begins with "D."

1. A round point
   A woman's name

   ANSWER _____

2. A fruit
   A couple goes on one

   ANSWER _____

3. An individual feature
   A small detachment of troops

   ANSWER _____

4. To call on a phone
   The face of a clock or watch

   ANSWER _____

5. To aim in a direction
   To speak clearly

   ANSWER _____

6. To become incorporated into a liquid
   To close down

   ANSWER _____

7. A product not made abroad
   An indoor pet

   ANSWER _____

8. A lower place
   A feeling

   ANSWER _____

9. To make lines and marks
   A tie

   ANSWER _____

10. To let fall
    A small portion of liquid

    ANSWER _____

11. To operate a car
    To urge to attain a goal

    ANSWER _____

12. Fine particles everywhere
    To cover lightly with a powder

    ANSWER _____

13. To politely refuse
    To become less

    ANSWER _____

14. To push into low position
    To make someone feel bad

    ANSWER _____

LANGUAGE

15. Lacking excitement

Not bright

ANSWER _____

16. To plunge steeply

To go headfirst

ANSWER _____

17. A quantity of medicine

A portion

ANSWER _____

18. A structure extending across a ship

To decorate festively

ANSWER _____

WORD MAZE – PATRIOTIC

Find your way through the maze by connecting letters to spell out words. Write the words on the next page. You may move forward, backward, up, or down, but no letters may be connected more than once.

START

R	F	N	R	W	Q	D	L	M	E	R	C
E	M	O	B	F	V	E	Y	K	P	D	O
E	D	I	L	S	E	C	E	P	L	E	D
W	O	T	A	R	A	L	C	H	W	E	G
A	M	I	N	D	E	P	N	O	D	A	E
D	E	C	P	P	C	E	E	N	K	L	R
U	W	I	I	L	S	N	D	G	E	L	V
T	Q	T	S	E	Q	L	K	I	C	B	Q
Y	V	E	U	J	E	C	N	A	U	Y	P
O	L	T	B	V	H	A	C	B	S	O	T
M	A	E	D	B	A	M	U	P	V	B	N
B	K	R	B	I	M	B	C	K	N	F	B
G	J	A	N	L	U	V	V	V	K	L	V

END

VISUAL–SPATIAL

WORDS

1. _____

2. _____

3. _____

4. _____

5. _____

6. _____

7. _____

8. _____

BETTING WORDS

The answer to each clue contains the letters "BET."

1. More pleasing or acceptable than something else

    ANSWER _____

2. Disloyal; to act in a way that is contrary to a promise made

    ANSWER _____

3. A frozen dessert made with fruit syrup and ice

    ANSWER _____

4. To and from; from one place to another

    ANSWER _____

5. Act of becoming engaged to marry someone

    ANSWER _____

6. All the letters used to represent a language

    ANSWER _____

7. A medical disorder producing excessive urine

    ANSWER _____

SHAPE MATCH 2

Circle the two matching shapes.

1

2

3

4

5   (row 5)

6   (row 6)

7

8

TRUE OR FALSE FACTS 2

Determine if each statement is True or False. Challenge yourself to answer as quickly as you can.

1. A customer serves the waitress.   True   False

2. Rinse with mouthwash to aid bad breath.   True   False

3. Mold can be used in making cheese.   True   False

4. Roses smell worse than cat litter.   True   False

5. Dehydration can cause delirium.   True   False

6. Golf requires less walking than Ping-Pong.   True   False

7. Dogs are never man's best friend.   True   False

8. Calculus is not as hard as basic math.   True   False

9. Jury trials are held in a courtroom.   True   False

10. Auctioneers rarely learn to talk fast.   True   False

11. A cotton shirt is not as warm as a wool jacket.   True   False

12. A plate will hold anything a bowl can hold.   True   False

13. Herbivores eat meat.   True   False

14. Botanists always study plants.   True   False

15. Toothpaste is sweeter than fudge.   True   False

16. Elbows are the largest joints in the body.   True   False

17. Hard-boiled eggs take more than 2 minutes to make.   True   False

PROCESSING SPEED

18. In math, multiplying two negatives equals a positive.　　True　　False

19. Every part of a true sentence must be true.　　True　　False

20. September is after March.　　True　　False

21. Cats love to take baths.　　True　　False

22. Thunder always comes before rain.　　True　　False

23. If yesterday was Wednesday, then tomorrow is Friday.　　True　　False

24. ½ never equals 50 percent.　　True　　False

MEMORY

MISMATCH 2

Pick out the one item that does not fit the category, and explain the *reason* why it does not fit.

1. Car, Jet Ski, Truck, Golf cart

   Mismatch item_____

   *Reason*_____

2. Shred, Cube, Mix, Slice

   Mismatch item_____

   *Reason*_____

3. Tenderloin, Ham, Strip, Sirloin

   Mismatch item_____

   *Reason*_____

4. Fountain, Steam, Ice, Droplets

   Mismatch item_____

   *Reason*_____

5. Lagoon, Waves, Lake, Swamp

   Mismatch item_____

   *Reason*_____

6. Aisle, Road, Stream, Sidewalk

   Mismatch item_____

   *Reason*_____

7. A pup, A joey, A sheep, A fawn

   Mismatch item_____

   *Reason*_____

8. Facts, Truth, Proof, Report

Mismatch item_____

*Reason*_____

9. Invention, Story, Reality, Fiction

Mismatch item_____

*Reason*_____

10. Manuscript, Pamphlet, Brochure, Flyer

Mismatch item_____

*Reason*_____

11. Emotion, Reaction, Answer, Sentiment

Mismatch item_____

*Reason*_____

12. Kinship, Branch, Relative, Tribe

Mismatch item_____

*Reason*_____

13. Ocean, Beach towel, Sunglasses, Sunblock

Mismatch item_____

*Reason*_____

14. Linebacker, Shortstop, Receiver, Kicker

Mismatch item_____

*Reason*_____

15. Pistol, Knife, Armor, Dart

Mismatch item_____

*Reason*_____

16. Oregon, Ohio, Seattle, Delaware

Mismatch item_____

*Reason*_____

17. Small, Microscope, Tiny, Miniscule

Mismatch item_____

*Reason*_____

WORDS FULL OF FUN

The answer to each clue contains the letters "FUN."

1. An activity or purpose natural to a person or thing

   ANSWER _____

2. A sum of money saved or made available for a particular purpose

   ANSWER _____

3. Spore-producing organisms feeding on organic matter

   ANSWER _____

4. A tube that is wide at the top and narrow at the bottom

   ANSWER _____

5. To pay back

   ANSWER _____

6. A ceremony to honor a person who passed away

   ANSWER _____

7. To fail to function normally

   ANSWER _____

WHAT'S THE CATEGORY? 4

Put these words into the most correct category.

menu	shells	booths	sheets
cashier	needles	wreckage	utensils
bandages	coral	medication	elevator
sand	insurance	divers	oil
spices	tide		

1. Things found in an ocean:

    _____   _____

    _____   _____

    _____

2. Things found in a hospital

    _____   _____

    _____   _____

    _____

3. Things found in a restaurant

    _____   _____

    _____   _____

    _____

WHAT'S NEXT? 2

Determine which shape comes next in the pattern.

1. [\ ] [^] ~ [^] [\ ] ~ [\ ] [

a. ^ b.] c. \

2. « « ¤ » » » « « ¤

a. « b. ¤ c. »

3. ʅ ʂ ƥ ɋ ʅ ʂ ƥ ɋ ʅ

a. ʂ b. ƥ c. ɋ

4. ‖ ǂ ǂ ¬ ± ‖ ǂ

a. ¬ b. ǂ c. ±

5. ð ø ö Ö Õ ð ø ö

a. Õ b. ð c. Ö

6. ɣ ƛ ƛ ƛ ƴ ƴ ɣ ɣ ƛ ƛ

a. ɣ b. ƛ c. ƴ

7. д Д Ѝ Ꜧ ħ ꜧ д Д Ѝ Ꜧ ħ

a. д b. ħ c. ꜧ

EXECUTIVE FUNCTIONING

CALCULATIONS

Calculate the correct answer for each question.

1. The sum total of all 10 of your grandchildrens' ages is 110. If they are all 2 years apart in age, what are their ages?

    ANSWER _____

2. While at Katy's ballet recital you see that the auditorium holds 240 people. Two-thirds of the seats are full. How many empty seats are open?

    ANSWER _____

3. You are putting away savings to go on a cruise. The cruise leaving November 1st costs $1,800. It is now February; how much do you have to save each month to afford the cruise?

    ANSWER _____

4. You have 24 yards of ribbon to wrap 8 presents. How much ribbon does each box get?

    ANSWER _____

5. You have to divide up your bowl of candy among your 6 grandchildren. The 3 oldest grandkids get four more pieces each than the younger ones. If there are 48 pieces of candy, how many pieces do the younger ones get?

    ANSWER _____

6. While building your porch steps, you determine that it takes 3 ¾ planks of wood to build one step. You want the staircase to be 8 steps. How many planks of wood do you need to buy?

    ANSWER _____

7. You are driving 57 miles per hour on the freeway. You want to get to Atlanta, which is 228 miles away. How long will it take you to get there?

    ANSWER _____

8. You are ordering dinner tables for a party of 70 people. The company you called said they have small tables that fit 5 people and large tables that fit 12 people. How many large and small tables should you order so that you have the exact amount of seating?

ANSWER _____

9. You are using your large coat closet to hold guests' coats during the party. When the party begins 4 coats are put in. Then 8 coats are put in and 2 taken out. Then 4 coats are put in before half of the coats in the closet are taken out. Finally, at the end of the night, 6 coats are taken out of the closet. How many coats are left inside the closet?

ANSWER _____

HOW MANY WORDS? 3

How many words can you make out of the letters in the two words below? You can rearrange the letters in any order you want and you do not have to use every letter in each new word.

1. Prestidigitation

2. Mellow

WORDS FULL OF INK

The answer to each clue contains the letters "INK."

1. To use your mind to actively form ideas

   ANSWER _____

2. A connection between two things

   ANSWER _____

3. To descend below the surface of a liquid

   ANSWER _____

4. To have a strong unpleasant odor

   ANSWER _____

5. A liquid to swallow

   ANSWER _____

6. To attempt to repair something in a casual way

   ANSWER _____

7. To make smaller in size

   ANSWER _____

8. A slight fold in something

   ANSWER _____

TWO-LETTER PLACEMENT 2

Choose which two-letter combo will make a word when added to the letters below.

al   ac   is   in   la   ca   si

1. c a n ____ e

2. ____ t u a l

3. d ____ c o

4. ____ l o w

5. i n ____ n d

6. ____ l m

7. f a ____ t

8. f ____ t o r

9. g o s ____ p

10. f l o r ____

11. ____ b o r

12. c r ____ p y

13. i n ____ d e

14. k ____ d l e

15. f o s ____ l

16. l o c ____

LANGUAGE

17. _____ _____ g n

18. _____ _____ s u e

19. d i _____ _____ o g u e

20. b _____ _____ n k

21. d e _____ _____ r e

22. l e g _____ _____

23. l o _____ _____ l

24. e n _____ _____ t

25. c o u _____ _____ n

26. s _____ _____ i v a

27. s _____ _____ r f

28. r a _____ _____ e

29. p _____ _____ q u e

30. g r a _____ _____

31. l _____ _____ e a r

32. f i s c _____ _____

33. r e _____ _____ t

34. w _____ _____ e

ORDERED NUMBERS 2

Pick the one statement that is CORRECT.

1. **53691**

A) 9 is right of 1.
B) 9 is between 3 and 1.
C) 5 is not first.
D) 6 is left of 3.

2. **74182**

A) 1 is not in the middle.
B) 4 is right of 1.
C) 8 is between 1 and 2.
D) 4 is third.

3. **64823**

A) 4 is right of 2.
B) 3 is left of 2.
C) 2 is between 6 and 8.
D) 8 is right of 6.

4. **91734**

A) 3 is between 4 and 7.
B) 9 is not first.
C) 7 is not in the middle.
D) 4 is left of 3.

5. **67928**

A) 2 is right of 8.
B) 6 is right of 9.
C) 8 is right of 7.
D) 8 is not last.

6. **35421**

A) 2 is between 3 and 4.
B) 5 is left of 3.
C) 4 is not in the middle.
D) 2 is fourth.

7. **65283**

A) 2 is after 8.
B) 5 is left of 6.
C) 8 is left of 5.
D) 5 is left of 2.

8. **57139**

A) 7 is between 1 and 9.
B) 3 is right of 1.
C) 1 is left of 5.
D) 1 is first.

EXECUTIVE FUNCTIONING

ORDERED SYMBOLS 1

Pick the one statement that is WRONG.

1.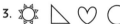

   A) Circle is before Triangle.
   B) Square is between Star and Arrow.
   C) Triangle is right of Arrow.
   D) Star is left of Circle.

2. ◇ + ☾ = 🛢

   A) Crescent is right of Plus.
   B) Diamond is left of Plus.
   C) Equals is before Cylinder.
   D) Cylinder is third.

3. ☼ ◺ ♡ ◯ ▭

   A) Sun is left of Heart.
   B) Rectangle is between Sun and Circle.
   C) Triangle is left of Heart.
   D) Circle is right of Triangle.

4. ⇨ △ 🛢 ♡ ◇

   A) Cylinder is between Heart and Arrow.
   B) Heart is fourth.
   C) Diamond is left of Heart.
   D) Arrow is not last.

5. 🛢 ☆ = + ◺

   A) Star is between Equals and Plus.
   B) Cylinder is left of Star.
   C) Plus is right of Star.
   D) Triangle is fifth.

6. ◯ ☾ ☼ △ ▭

   A) Crescent is left of Sun.
   B) Triangle is between Sun and Circle.
   C) Rectangle is right of Triangle.
   D) Circle is left of Crescent.

7. ☐ △ ▭ ◇ ♡

   A) Diamond is right of Triangle.
   B) Triangle is between Square and Rectangle.
   C) Heart is right of Diamond.
   D) Rectangle is second.

8. = ☾ ⇨ ☆ +

   A) Star is between Arrow and Plus.
   B) Crescent is left of Arrow.
   C) Star is right of Arrow.
   D) Plus is left of Star.

THREE-LETTER PLACEMENT 2

Choose which three-letter combo will make a word when added to the letters below.

ous   ear   ran   tar   ker   nor   cue

1. e n d ___ ___ ___

2. t a r ___ ___ ___

3. s p ___ ___ ___ e

4. w a l ___ ___ ___

5. b ___ ___ ___ d

6. c l ___ ___ ___

7. h ___ ___ ___ e

8. a l ___ ___ ___

9. h o ___ ___ ___

10. b ___ ___ ___ i n g

11. e r ___ ___ ___ d

12. c a l l ___ ___ ___

13. s e e ___ ___ ___

14. s ___ ___ ___ t

15. ___ ___ ___ t h

16. o ___ ___ ___ g e

LANGUAGE

17. w ___ ___ ___ y

18. f u r i ___ ___ ___

19. ___ ___ ___ n e l

20. h ___ ___ ___ t

21. s ___ ___ ___ e

22. ___ ___ ___ d

23. g ___ ___ ___ d

24. r e s ___ ___ ___

25. s e r i ___ ___ ___

26. ___ ___ ___ t h

27. b a ___ ___ ___ s

28. s ___ ___ ___ c h

29. b a r b e ___ ___ ___

30. r o c ___ ___ ___

31. u n l ___ ___ ___ n

32. l ___ ___ ___ y

33. c ___ ___ ___ k y

34. s ___ ___ ___ s

ASKING WORDS

The answer to each clue contains the letters "ASK."

1. A face covering to hide identity

   ANSWER _____

2. A small flat container for alcohol

   ANSWER _____

3. A job assigned to somebody

   ANSWER _____

4. Off center or at an angle

   ANSWER _____

5. A woven container with a handle

   ANSWER _____

6. A rubber seal used to render a joint impermeable to gas or liquid

   ANSWER _____

LANGUAGE

MATCHING CLUES 5

Match two of the word-parts to make a word that fits the clue. Each word-part is used only once.

abr   cab   upt   lad

abs   bal   orb   le

1. _____ a thick rope of wire

   _____ to soak up

   _____ sudden; unexpected

   _____ a song narrating a story

bar   bad   bal   dou

let   ger   ble   ely

2. _____ to pester

   _____ a formal artistic dance

   _____ to almost not

   _____ twice as many

LANGUAGE

SHARED NATURE LETTERS

Write in a letter that completes each word so that a nature word reads down.

1. w a i ____
   c ____ a s h
   l ____ a d
   ____ a s y

2. f i ____ e r
  o b ____ y
   l ____ u g h
  ____ a l l
  c ____ a p e l

3. s ____ i n g
  n ____ g h t
  k i ____ g
  ____ a r t

4. s t a ____ e
   g ____ a r
   l e ____ p
   e ____ e n
   n ____ a r
  ____ o l d

5. s ____ u g
  ____ l l e y
  ____ i n d
   r ____ a d

6. c a ____ e
  s o u ____
   r ____ a d
  ____ a l k
  k e ____ p
   t ____ y

7. c a ____ e l
   c ____ l a
  ____ s e
  ____ a m e
  s p i ____
  ____ i r
   l ____ t e r
  c o i ____

8. ____ e l t
  ____ a i n
   h ____ a r t
   v ____ i n
   g a ____ e
   t r u ____

9. s u p e ____
   b e ____ r d
   h ____ d e
   l e ____ d

WORDS FULL OF AIR 1

The answer to each clue contains the letters "AIR."

1. A finger-shaped cream pastry

    ANSWER _____

2. A feeling of hopelessness

    ANSWER _____

3. Chief presiding officer of a company board

    ANSWER _____

4. A device to spray paint

    ANSWER _____

5. A treeless grass-covered US plain

    ANSWER _____

6. A card game for one

    ANSWER _____

7. To weaken something; to lessen the quality or strength

    ANSWER _____

8. A wealthy person whose net worth is more than a million dollars

    ANSWER _____

CALCULATION WORD PROBLEMS 3

1. You head out for a walk at 9:15 and walk for 75 minutes. What time do you arrive back home?

    _____

2. You are finished shopping at the grocery store and walk to the checkout registers. You have 2 boxes of granola bars, a gallon of milk, a canister of coffee, coffee filters, tea bags, a pound of sugar, and 3 boxes of cereal. Can you go in the express lane that says 15 items or fewer?

    _____

3. You take your grandchildren to a local park. There are 35 kids playing at the park today. If there are 16 more kids than adults, how many adults are there at the park today?

    _____

4. You count 14 red flowers and 18 yellow flowers in your garden. The next morning when you wake up and go outside, you see that 3 red flowers died and 2 yellow flowers died, but you see 6 more flowers that bloomed overnight. Now, how many total flowers do you have in your garden?

    _____

5. You are having family over and want to buy enough sodas for everyone to have one and then have some left over for yourself for one week. There will be 4 adults and 3 kids plus you and your spouse. You drink one soda each day. How many sodas will you have to buy?

    _____

6. You are making flyers for your 32 club members to advertise the fund-raiser. You want each person to take and hand out 20 flyers. How many copies of the flyer should you make?

    _____

CALCULATION

"G" WORDS

Using two clues, fill in the correct word that begins with "G."

1. Soccer's posts and net

   The object of your effort

   ANSWER _____

2. Happy

   Pleased

   ANSWER _____

3. A form of play or sport

   To manipulate

   ANSWER _____

4. Simple elegance

   Unmerited favor

   ANSWER _____

5. A person invited to your home

   Company

   ANSWER _____

6. To prepare someone for a particular purpose

   To brush a horse

   ANSWER _____

7. A diagram

   To plot and measure variables

   ANSWER _____

8. A metal cooker used outside

   To question intensely

   ANSWER _____

9. To watch over

   Worn to prevent injury

   ANSWER _____

10. Disgusting

    Without tax

    ANSWER _____

MATCH THE PARTS 2

Match a word-part on the left with a word-part on the right to form a word and write it on the line. You can use each word-part only once.

1. beh   ive   _____

     got   ors   _____

     loc   ors   _____

     rum   ten   _____

     fla   ave   _____

     mot   vor   _____

     par   ody   _____

     col   ket   _____

2. the   nel   _____

     wor   ble   _____

     bun   ory   _____

     dev   dle   _____

     fun   nce   _____

     inj   ker   _____

     nua   our   _____

     hum   ure   _____

OUR WORDS

The answer to each clue contains the letters "OUR."

1. The business of providing information to people visiting places of interest

ANSWER _____

2. An attractive quality that makes certain people seem appealing or special

ANSWER _____

3. A place, person, or thing from which something comes or can be obtained

ANSWER _____

4. Act of traveling from one place to another

ANSWER _____

5. Presided over by a judge

ANSWER _____

6. Taste and enjoy it completely

ANSWER _____

7. Postpone a meeting

ANSWER _____

8. A messenger who transports goods or documents

ANSWER _____

9. A connoisseur of good food with a discerning palate

ANSWER _____

PLACEMENT OF LETTERS 2

Choose a word-part from the left and fit it into letters on the right to make a word.

 You can use each word-part only once.

1. gn

  ng

  an

  en

  gi

  ng

  ld

  ya

ch ___ ___ ge

ag ___ ___ cy

re ___ ___ on

to ___ ___ ue

fi ___ ___ er

ma ___ ___ et

vo ___ ___ ge

go ___ ___ en

2. no

  go

  ng

  si

  gh

  al

  go

  gn

di ___ ___ ogue

hi ___ ___ er

si ___ ___ al

ig ___ ___ re

vi ___ ___ r

as ___ ___ gn

wa ___ ___ ns

mi ___ ___ le

LANGUAGE

3. og   ga _____ _____ op

ri   be _____ _____ ng

ge   or _____ _____ ge

ow   cr _____ _____ ch

ll   du _____ _____ ng

lo   sl _____ _____ an

un   gr _____ _____ th

an   le _____ _____ nd

4. rb   en _____ _____ ne

ig   ti _____ _____ ng

ci   ge _____ _____ le

gi   ha _____ _____ or

vi   br _____ _____ ht

ig   or _____ _____ in

nt   ra _____ _____ ng

mi   lo _____ _____ ng

SOLUTIONS TO A PROBLEM

Describe two different ways to solve these problems. There is not one right answer, so be as creative as you like.

Feeling stressed out 1. _____
2. _____

Car won't start 1. _____
2. _____

Can't find keys 1. _____
2. _____

Have a headache 1. _____
2. _____

Late bill payment 1. _____
2. _____

Electricity goes out 1. _____
2. _____

Burn your hand 1. _____
2. _____

A fly in the kitchen 1. _____
2. _____

Neighbor's dog won't stop barking 1. _____
2. _____

Lost your wallet 1. _____
2. _____

Double-booked appointments 1. _____
2. _____

Locked keys in car 1. _____
2. _____

Squeaky door hinge 1. _____
2. _____

REASONING

ORDERED SYMBOLS 2

Pick the one statement that is CORRECT.

1. 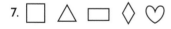 ☆ ○ □ △ ⇨

   A) Circle is right of Triangle.
   B) Square is between Star and Circle.
   C) Triangle is right of Square.
   D) Star is right of Circle.

2. ◇ + ☾ = ⬭

   A) Crescent is left of Plus.
   B) Diamond is left of Equals.
   C) Equals is right of Cylinder.
   D) Cylinder is fourth.

3. ☼ ◺ ♡ ○ ▭

   A) Triangle is right of Rectangle.
   B) Circle is between Sun and Heart.
   C) Heart is not in the middle.
   D) Sun is left of Triangle.

4. ⇨ △ ⬭ ♡ ◇

   A) Cylinder is right of Arrow.
   B) Heart is third.
   C) Diamond is left of Heart.
   D) Arrow is not first.

5. ⬭ ☆ = + ◺

   A) Star is right of Plus.
   B) Cylinder is right of Star.
   C) Plus is right of Star.
   D) Equals is fourth.

6. ○ ☾ ☼ △ ▭

   A) Crescent is right of Rectangle.
   B) Triangle is between Sun and Circle.
   C) Sun is left of Crescent.
   D) Circle is left of Triangle.

7. □ △ ▭ ◇ ♡

   A) Diamond is not fourth.
   B) Triangle is right of Rectangle.
   C) Rectangle is left of Square.
   D) Heart is right of Diamond.

8. = ☾ ⇨ ☆ +

   A) Star is between Arrow and Equals.
   B) Crescent is left of Star.
   C) Plus is left of Arrow.
   D) Equals is right of Crescent.

WORDS THAT HAM IT UP 1

The answer to each clue contain the letters "HAM."

1. A lizard that changes color

    ANSWER _____

2. A sweet plain type of brown cracker

    ANSWER _____

3. A pounding tool

    ANSWER _____

4. Something fake that is presented as genuine

    ANSWER _____

5. To make movement or progress difficult

    ANSWER _____

6. A hair-cleaning product

    ANSWER _____

7. A meeting place of legislature or court

    ANSWER _____

8. A hanging bed made of canvas or netting

    ANSWER _____

LANGUAGE

COMPOUND WORDS 2

Make at least three compound words with these beginnings.

1. Bed _____ _____ _____

2. News _____ _____ _____

3. Lady _____ _____ _____

4. Pig _____ _____ _____

5. Hand _____ _____ _____

6. Life _____ _____ _____

7. Sand _____ _____ _____

8. Fire _____ _____ _____

9. Eye _____ _____ _____

10. Thumb _____ _____ _____

11. Rain _____ _____ _____

12. Moon _____ _____ _____

13. Butter _____ _____ _____

14. Book _____ _____ _____

15. Door _____ _____ _____

16. Head _____ _____ _____

MEMORY

SEQUENCING ITEMS 3

Discover a logical way to sequence these items, and explain the reason why you put them in that order. No alphabetical order allowed.

1. Algebra, Calculus, Geometry, Trigonometry

    1st _____ 2nd _____ 3rd _____ 4th _____

    Reason _____

2. Marilyn Monroe, Rosie the Riveter, *The Tramp*, *I Love Lucy*

    1st _____ 2nd _____ 3rd _____ 4th _____

    Reason _____

3. Moon landing, Amelia Earhart, Berlin Wall torn down, United Nations founded

    1st _____ 2nd _____ 3rd _____ 4th _____

    Reason _____

4. Orange, Black, Yellow, Blue

    1st _____ 2nd _____ 3rd _____ 4th _____

    Reason _____

5. Reading a brochure, Running a marathon, Dialing a phone number, Writing a novel

    1st _____ 2nd _____ 3rd _____ 4th _____

    Reason _____

6. Put in mailbox, Stamp, Write letter, Address envelope

    1st _____ 2nd _____ 3rd _____ 4th _____

    Reason _____

7. Light match, Stack firewood, Dig hole, Gather kindling

    1st _____ 2nd _____ 3rd _____ 4th _____

    Reason _____

8. Belt, Shoes, Pants, Socks

1st _____ 2nd _____ 3rd _____ 4th _____

Reason _____

9. Water, Dig hole, Cover with dirt, Place seed

1st _____ 2nd _____ 3rd _____ 4th _____

Reason _____

10. Constructing, Planning, Buying supplies, Designing

1st _____ 2nd _____ 3rd _____ 4th _____

Reason _____

11. Running, Jogging, Walking, Sprinting

1st _____ 2nd _____ 3rd _____ 4th _____

Reason _____

12. Anniversary, Courting, Vows, Reception

1st _____ 2nd _____ 3rd _____ 4th _____

Reason _____

13. Los Angeles, New York, Boston, Nashville

1st _____ 2nd _____ 3rd _____ 4th _____

Reason _____

14. Thanksgiving, Halloween, Valentine's Day, Labor Day

1st _____ 2nd _____ 3rd _____ 4th _____

Reason _____

15. Change, Receipt, Pay, Choose

1st _____ 2nd _____ 3rd _____ 4th _____

Reason _____

MISSPELLED WORDS 2

Pick out the words that are misspelled words, and correct their spelling.

acceptible	_____	acomodate	_____
liason	_____	occasionally	_____
exhilarat	_____	personnel	_____
maneuver	_____	pastime	_____
receit	_____	guarranttee	_____
harass	_____	sargent	_____
greatful	_____	accidentally	_____
independent	_____	threshole	_____
miniscule	_____	humerous	_____
consensus	_____	ignorence	_____
lisenc	_____	milinium	_____
restaurant	_____	existence	_____
jewlry	_____	fiery	_____
rymth	_____	priority	_____

TWO COMMON LETTERS 4

Scan each line to find the two letters each word has in common. The letters are next to each other. Challenge yourself to go as quickly as you can.

Example: bounce and balance both have "ce"

COMMON LETTERS

1. although   fight   higher   ghost   laugh   _____

2. calmer   ailment   filmed   mailman   almond   _____

3. basket   bearskin   outskirt   sketch   masking   _____

4. afraid   carefree   frowning   unfreeze   suffrage   _____

5. billable   backstab   reasonable   abstract   laborer   _____

6. butcher   fabulous   abundant   tabulate   debutant   _____

7. artistic   bruising   discern   baptism   finished   _____

8. assembly   amenable   dribble   humble   crucible   _____

9. banished   cheapen   coherent   heavenly   mustache   _____

10. conjured   justice   reinjured   adjunct   perjury   _____

BLANK CROSSWORD

Fill in the crossword with your own words. There is no one right answer.

LANGUAGE

MATCHING CLUES 6

Match two of the word-parts to make a word that fits the clue. Each word-part is used only once.

edi	bel	ble	ore
ong	bef	ble	hum

1.
_____ preceding

_____ to be in the rightful place

_____ fit to eat

_____ modest

bon	bor	la	ain
obt	mar	rib	ble

2.
_____ to work hard

_____ a ball of colored glass

_____ to acquire

_____ narrow strips of fabric

WORDS WITH OUT

The answer to each clue contains the letters "OUT."

1. A sequence of actions regularly followed

   ANSWER _____

2. To put forth shoots of a plant

   ANSWER _____

3. To utter a loud call or cry

   ANSWER _____

4. A way directed along a specified course

   ANSWER _____

5. The projecting nose and mouth of an animal

   ANSWER _____

6. The period between childhood and adult age

   ANSWER _____

7. Money given as compensation or a dividend

   ANSWER _____

8. A person sent out ahead of a main force to gather information

   ANSWER _____

9. A small store selling fashionable clothes or accessories

   ANSWER _____

LANGUAGE

PARTS OF A WHAT? 1

Put these words into the most correct category.

lens window rudder cord
deck ignition shutter receiver
speaker flash hood aperture
keypad wheel masthead tiller

1. Parts of a camera

   _____   _____

   _____   _____

2. Parts of a phone

   _____   _____

   _____   _____

3. Parts of a car

   _____   _____

   _____   _____

4. Parts of a boat

   _____   _____

   _____   _____

WHAT'S THAT PHRASE? 2

Fill in the letters to complete the familiar phrase. There is a clue to help.

1. E __ __ __ Y C __ __ __ D H __ __ __
   S __ __ __ R L __ __ __ __ G
   To be optimistic even in difficult times

2. F __ __ H O __ __ O __ W __ __ __ R
   Someone in a situation they are unfamiliar with or unsuited for

3. G __ F __ __ B __ __ __ E
   To risk it all

4. G __ O __ __ O __ A L __ __ __
   To put yourself in a risky situation to help someone

5. G __ __ __ Y T __ __ - S __ __ __ __
   A smugly virtuous person

6. H __ __ __ __ __ A __ A C __ __ __ __
   A state of being delighted

7. H __ __ D P __ __ L T __ S __ __ __ __ __ W
   Something that is difficult to accept

8. H __ __ __ O __ __ __ H __ __ __ __
   Fall deeply in love

9. I __ __ __ P __ __ __ __ __ __
   To be in a difficult situation

MEMORY

10. J ___ ___ ___ - ___ ___ -A ___ ___ -T ___ ___ ___ ___ S

To have skill in multiple trades

11. J ___ ___ ___ T ___ ___ G ___ ___

When something happens too early; starting too soon

12. K ___ ___ P O ___ T ___ ___ ___ ___ ___ N'

To press forward, not stop

13. K ___ ___ ___ ___ Y ___ ___ ___ S ___ ___ ___ ___ O ___ ___

To be taken by surprise

14. A M ___ ___ ___ ___ ___ ___ ___ O ___ ___ O ___ ___

M ___ ___ ___ ___ ___ ___ ___

To escalate a small thing and turn it into a big problem

15. M ___ C ___ ___ O ___ T ___ ___

Something you find delightful

16. O ___ C ___ ___ ___ ___ N ___ ___ ___

Strong feelings of happiness and satisfaction

17. R ___ ___ ___ O ___ Y ___ ___ ___ P ___ ___ ___ ___ ___

To spoil someone's fun

LETTER TRANSFER 4

Fill in the word(s) to answer the clue, then transfer those numbered letters to the lines on the next page for the final message.

1. Elephant tusks are made out of this material

   _____ _____ _____ _____ _____
    1   2   3   4   5

2. This is the hardest substance known

   _____ _____ _____ _____ _____ _____ _____
    6   1   7   8   3   9   6

3. The last name of the second man on the moon

   _____ _____ _____ _____ _____ _____
    7   10   6   4   1   9

4. The Grand Canyon is in this state

   _____ _____ _____ _____ _____ _____ _____
    7   4   1   11   3   9   7

5. The name of the cartoon starring Charlie Brown

   _____ _____ _____ _____ _____ _____ _____
    12   13   7   9   14   15   16

MEMORY

6. The country where reggae music originated

17	7	8	7	1	18	7

7. The sport in which you would use a "sand iron"

19	3	10	20

FINAL MESSAGE:

```
____ ____ ____    ____ ____    ____  q____ ____ ____ ____ ____ ____ ____   ____ ____
 7   19   13    1   16    7      14   13   16   15    1    3    9     3    20

____ ____ ____ ____    ____ ____ ____ ____    ____ ____ ____ ____ ____  :
 8    1    9    6     3    2   13    4      8    7   15   15   13    4

____ ____    ____ ____ ____    ____ ____ ____    ____    ____ ____ ____ ____ ,
 1   20     5    3   14     6    3    9     15      8    1    9    6

____ ____ ____    ____ ____ ____    ____ ____ ____ ____ ____ .
 7   19   13     6    3    9     15     8    7   15   15   13    4
```

COMPLETE THE WORD SEARCH 2

First fill in the answers to the clues, then find those words in the word search grid.

The first letter and number of letters in the word are given.

1. To secretly get married   E ___ ___ ___ ___

2. Dried grass   H ___ ___

3. To give to a charity   D ___ ___ ___ ___ ___

4. A doorway is an   E ___ ___ ___ ___ ___ ___

5. You inherit these   G ___ ___ ___ ___

6. To not listen to someone speaking   I ___ ___ ___ ___ ___

7. To calm and train a horse   T ___ ___ ___

8. A penny   C ___ ___ ___

9. A large spoon you use to serve soup   L ___ ___ ___ ___

10. Formal choirs wear these   R ___ ___ ___ ___

COMPLETE THE WORD SEARCH 2

Words can be in any direction.

```
A  W  L  B  Q  R  M  T  H  E  P  R  A  L
D  F  Y  O  G  B  K  L  A  D  L  E  Q  Y
T  S  S  K  E  L  N  O  J  E  N  H  G  S
W  A  L  F  N  L  I  S  D  S  R  E  W  L
A  R  M  T  E  R  O  B  E  S  E  R  A  M
H  P  K  E  S  P  L  P  H  O  N  D  H  K
L  L  T  C  S  T  U  E  E  C  T  H  L  T
Q  H  A  Y  N  E  T  G  P  E  R  B  E  A
J  A  N  E  L  A  O  C  T  R  A  R  J  N
O  V  C  T  N  B  N  A  S  N  O  O  C
M  B  U  O  A  N  P  S  M  N  C  B  M  U
B  I  D  B  M  I  G  N  O  R  E  F  B  C
G  L  V  V  U  C  E  I  Y  K  J  L  G  V
```

UPSIDE DOWN

Determine which image is the original image upside down.

1. ANSWER _____

a.　　　b.　　　c.　　　d.

2. ANSWER _____

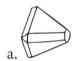

a.　　　b.　　　c.　　　d.

3. ANSWER _____

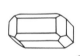 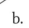

a.　　　b.　　　c.　　　d.

4. ANSWER _____

 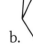

a.　　　b.　　　c.　　　d.

VISUAL–SPATIAL

HOT WORDS

The answer to each clue contains the letters "HOT."

1. An image produced on light-sensitive film

   ANSWER _____

2. A place for overnight stays

   ANSWER _____

3. An injection of a medicine

   ANSWER _____

4. A direct telephone link to a service, often available 24-7

   ANSWER _____

5. A small Y-shaped weapon used to propel objects

   ANSWER _____

6. The science of medical devices such as braces

   ANSWER _____

7. A person who has lost contact with reality

   ANSWER _____

8. A division into two groups of contradictory things

   ANSWER _____

LANGUAGE

LETTER-NUMBER SUBSTITUTION CODE 2

Using the code key, determine what words the numbers are spelling.

CODE KEY

A = 4   D = 92   U = 34   R = 23   O = 52

B = 19   E = 71   P = 87   S = 38   N = 96

C = 55   I = 26   L = 63   T = 45   V = 12

1. 4 87 87 63 26 55 4 19 63 71

WORD: _____

2. 87 23 4 55 45 26 55 71

WORD: _____

3. 71 23 4 92 26 55 4 45 71

WORD: _____

4. 23 71 87 63 26 55 4 45 71

WORD: _____

5. 92 71 38 87 26 55 4 19 63 71

WORD: _____

6. 87 23 71 92 26 55 45 4 19 63 71

WORD: _____

7. 71 92 34 55 4 45 26 52 96

WORD: _____

8. 4 63 63 52 55 4 45 71

WORD: _____

9. 23 71 12 52 55 4 19 63 71

WORD: _____

10. 55 4 19 26 96 71 45

WORD: _____

TWO DEFINITIONS 4

Two definitions for the same word are given. Fill in the correct word that matches both definitions.

1. A boat's standing area

   A stack of cards

   ANSWER _____

2. Not heavy

   Shines bright

   ANSWER _____

3. To sway back and forth

   Larger than a pebble

   ANSWER _____

4. Employees

   A walking stick

   ANSWER _____

5. Students receive these

   Levels of rank or value

   ANSWER _____

6. A short letter

   A musical component

   ANSWER _____

7. The answer after subtracting two numbers

   The quality that makes one thing unlike another

   ANSWER _____

8. The task of cleaning a fish to eat

   A tool to measure weight

   ANSWER _____

FIRST AND LAST LETTERS 3

Fill in the correct letters to make a word that matches the definition.

1. ___ antru ___   a burst of bad temper

2. ___ ola ___   a type of eclipse

3. ___ tla ___   a book of maps

4. ___ ea ___   to show the way

5. ___ ear ___   listened to

6. ___ eig ___   a royal rule

7. ___ bov ___   over

8. ___ ati ___   a silky smooth fabric

9. ___ in ___   fishing string

10. ___ is ___   an aspiration

11. ___ tai ___   a laundry problem

12. ___ ro ___   to let fall

CALENDAR QUIZ 4

Use the calendar clues to determine the correct date.

SUNDAY	MONDAY	TUESDAY	WEDNESDAY	THURSDAY	FRIDAY	SATURDAY
	1	2	3	4	5	6
7	8	9	10	11	12	13
14	15	16	17	18	19	20
21	22	23	24	25	26	27
28	29	30	31			

1. This date is in the last week of the month.

    It is on a weekend.

    What is the date? _____

2. This date is on a weekday.

    It is not a single digit.

    It is on a Friday.

    It does not begin with a 1.

    What is the date? _____

EXECUTIVE FUNCTIONING

3. This date is between the 2nd and the 19th .

   It is on a weekend.

   It is not in the first weekend of the month.

   It is not the 14th.

   What is the date? _____

4. This date is not in the first half of the month.

   It is not in the middle of the week.

   It begins with a 3.

   What is the date? _____

RAPPING WORDS

The answer to each clue contains the letters "RAP."

1. A device designed to allow entry but not exit

ANSWER _____

2. To cover in paper or material

ANSWER _____

3. A strip of material with a buckle used to secure or carry something

ANSWER _____

4. Happening in a short time or at a fast pace

ANSWER _____

5. To arrange cloth loosely or casually around something

ANSWER _____

6. To push or pull a hard, sharp implement across a surface to remove matter

ANSWER _____

7. To deceive or trick

ANSWER _____

8. Relating to visual art

ANSWER _____

LANGUAGE

ONE COMMON LETTER 1

Scan each line to find the one letter each word has in common. Challenge yourself to go as quickly as you can.

Example: baker and milk both have "k"

					COMMON LETTER
1. accept	baptize	chirp	group	hippo	_____
2. sedan	adult	bends	blonde	tuned	_____
3. grump	bluff	church	aunt	menu	_____
4. radium	sermon	amazed	compass	manure	_____
5. parlor	Velcro	zealot	wallet	uphold	_____
6. entice	gothic	jockey	launch	peace	_____
7. abysmal	boyish	clingy	gypsy	hymnal	_____
8. jacket	banker	drunk	knife	parked	_____
9. finish	mashed	north	phlegm	school	_____
10. before	effect	faithful	softer	toffee	_____

MIDDLE LETTERS 3

Fill in the correct letters to make a word that matches the definition.

1. p _____ _____ a   an earnest request

2. n _____ _____ e   kind

3. t _____ _____ t   a camp shelter

4. i _____ _____ _____ r   not outer

5. a _____ _____ _____ e   an orchard fruit

6. m _____ _____ _____ c   to imitate

7. n _____ _____ _____ _____ e   to deny

8. l _____ _____ e   fishing bait

9. t _____ _____ _____ e   not those

10. c _____ _____ _____ l   infants do this

11. p _____ _____ _____ l   a bicycle part

12. t _____ _____ d   a warty amphibian

LANGUAGE

MEMORY CROSSWORD 2

First, spend two minutes studying the words in this crossword. Then turn the page for a quiz.

```
                    D
A   C   C   R   U   E
M                   T
O           M   A   R   K   E   R
E                   I
B   U   S   H   E   L
A       I
        N
        G
```

MEMORY CROSSWORD 2

(DON'T LOOK AT THIS PAGE UNTIL YOU'VE STUDIED PREVIOUS PAGE.)

Now look at the list of words below and circle the words that were in the crossword on the previous page.

MARKER

PALE

GATOR

ACCRUE

AMOEBA

PROTON

MERRY

OFFICE

DETAIL

GARDEN

BUSHEL

SING

PRIZE

IMAGES MEMORY 3

First, spend two minutes studying the images. Then turn the page for a quiz.

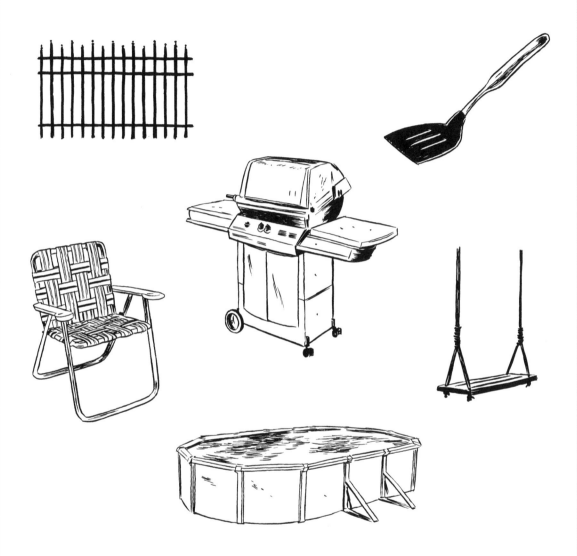

IMAGES MEMORY 3

(DON'T LOOK AT THIS PAGE UNTIL YOU'VE STUDIED PREVIOUS PAGE.)

Now look at the list of words below and circle the words that were images on the previous page.

SWING

SLIDE

TREE HOUSE

POOL

FENCE

GRILLED CHICKEN

SUNSCREEN

LAWN CHAIR

SPATULA

GARDEN

SHRUBS

BARBECUE GRILL

TOYS

NEIGHBOR

CALCULATION WORD PROBLEMS 4

1. A. You are painting bird houses to sell at a craft fair booth. You bought 15 bird houses that cost $6.98 each (no tax), and the paint costs $27 (no tax). How much does each bird house cost to make?

   _____

   B. You want to make a profit on the birdhouses. If you sell them for $25 each, how much profit would you make on each birdhouse?

   _____

   C. If you sell all 15 birdhouses, how much total profit would you make?

   _____

2. A group of 4 friends go picking strawberries at a farm field. Each basket holds 8 strawberries and each friend brings back 3 baskets. How many total strawberries does the group have?

   _____

3. There were 562 people at the county fair when it started raining. Half of them went home and 24 waited in their cars to see if the rain would stop. How many people stayed outside to enjoy the county fair despite the rain?

   _____

4. A museum reports that 214 tickets were sold ahead of time for an art exhibit, but half of those people brought a friend with them to see the exhibit too and bought their tickets at the door. How many total people came to see the art exhibit?

   _____

5. Your grandson saved up 562 pennies to buy toys at the toy store. He wants to buy 6 army men that cost $0.85 each. Does he have enough money?

   _____

WORDS FULL OF AIR 2

The answer to each clue contains the letters "AIR."

1. A series of steps

   ANSWER _____

2. Strands growing on a head or body

   ANSWER _____

3. A small imaginary creature with magical powers

   ANSWER _____

4. Not equal or just

   ANSWER _____

5. A farm for milk production

   ANSWER _____

6. Two similar things used together

   ANSWER _____

7. An event or occurrence that is known about; a social event

   ANSWER _____

8. To fix or mend something

   ANSWER _____

MATCHING CLUES 7

Match two of the word-parts to make a word that fits the clue. Each word-part is used only once.

lev   par   pat   en

ent   tree   el   ade

1. _____ a formal procession

   _____ a type of leather

   _____ smooth

   _____ main dish

ket   ase   no   er

eal   bas   te   id

2. _____ wicker carrier

   _____ rub out a mark

   _____ a quick letter

   _____ perfect

EDIT THE WORD 2

In the first column, change one letter in the original word to make a new word. In the second column, take out one letter from the original word and keep the rest of the letters in the same order to form a new word.

For example:

	CHANGE ONE LETTER	**TAKE OUT ONE LETTER**
Spank	Spark	Sank

		CHANGE ONE LETTER	**TAKE OUT ONE LETTER**
1.	Dusty		
2.	Farm		
3.	Rear		
4.	Shut		
5.	Fast		
6.	What		
7.	Here		
8.	Pair		

LANGUAGE

WHO IS THIS PERSON?

Determine the name of the person described by the clues.

1. This singer won an Oscar for
    From Here to Eternity in 1954 _____

2. This doctor wrote *The Common Sense Book
    of Baby and Child Care* _____

3. This political figure gave his "Iron Curtain" speech in 1946 _____

4. This author published his book *1984* in 1949 _____

5. This woman refused to give up her seat on a bus in 1955 _____

6. This film director released *Psycho* in 1960 _____

7. This president gave "The Man on the Moon" speech _____

8. This artist exhibited his piece *Campbell Soup Can* in 1962 _____

9. This talk-show host took over *The Tonight Show* in 1962 _____

10. This political figure gave a speech titled "I Have a Dream" _____

11. This man became the first African-American
    US Supreme Court Justice _____

12. This American man was the first man on the moon _____

13. In 1974, this president was the first ever to resign _____

14. This TV mogul established CNN in 1980 _____

15. This actor starred in *Rebel Without a Cause* in 1955 _____

MEMORY

TWO COMMON LETTERS 5

Scan each line to find the two letters each word has in common. The letters are next to each other. Challenge yourself to go as quickly as you can.

Example: bounce and balance both have "ce"

COMMON LETTERS

1. allows	floats	blooms	clowns	locker	_____
2. alumni	solemn	hymnal	columns	gymnast	_____
3. fabric	hubris	abroad	rubric	bruise	_____
4. chewed	flower	glowed	skewer	towels	_____
5. mildly	holder	seldom	yield	remold	_____
6. gothic	behind	orchid	hinges	rhinos	_____
7. whiskers	sketch	asking	frisky	risked	_____
8. charge	margin	purged	target	argyle	_____
9. protect	bootleg	brother	denote	idiotic	_____
10. buckle	attack	clocks	pocket	unpack	_____

PROCESSING SPEED

SHAPE MATCH 3

Circle the two matching shapes.

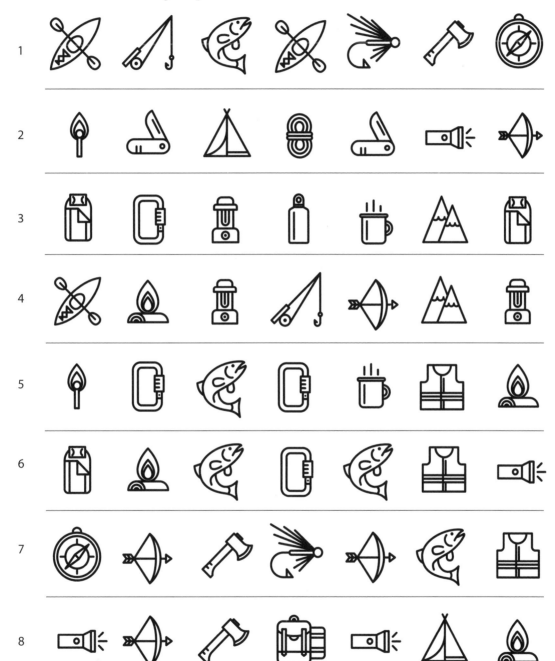

VISUAL–SATIAL

WORD MAZE – NEWS

Find your way through the maze by connecting letters to spell out words.
Write the words on the next page. You may move forward, backward, up, or down,
but no letters may be connected more than once.

START

A	P	T	R	W	Q	H	L	M	E	R	B
D	M	C	B	F	V	E	Y	K	P	D	O
G	N	O	L	S	E	A	S	N	E	H	K
W	R	S	J	K	H	D	L	I	S	E	F
A	E	S	E	R	P	N	M	U	A	R	T
H	P	B	P	P	C	H	K	L	O	D	I
L	O	R	T	L	S	S	T	U	C	H	C
Q	Q	G	E	E	Q	P	A	G	E	B	L
J	R	C	R	A	L	T	N	O	R	F	E
O	L	N	L	V	F	A	C	B	S	O	T
M	A	S	O	B	A	M	U	P	V	B	N
B	K	P	C	I	M	B	C	K	N	F	B
G	J	C	A	L	U	V	V	V	K	L	V

END

WORDS

1. ....

2. ....

3. ....

4. ....

5. ....

6. ....

7. ....

8. ....

PARTS OF A WHAT? 2

Put these words into the most correct category.

path attic   desks   wings
fertilizer cockpit notebooks motor
pantry rules   passengers sunshine
staircase rulers   fountain foyer

1. Parts of a house

_____ _____

_____ _____

2. Parts of a classroom

_____ _____

_____ _____

3. Parts of an airplane

_____ _____

_____ _____

4. Parts of a garden

_____ _____

_____ _____

REASONING

WORDS THAT HAM IT UP 2

The answer to each clue contains the letters "HAM."

1. A small rodent with cheek pouches

   ANSWER _____

2. Negative emotion; state of disgrace

   ANSWER _____

3. A white sparkling wine for special occasions

   ANSWER _____

4. A patty of ground meat

   ANSWER _____

5. A dried flower head used to make an herbal tea

   ANSWER _____

6. Disorganized failure; a state of messy disorder

   ANSWER _____

7. Supreme victor in a contest

   ANSWER _____

8. Leg tendon

   ANSWER _____

LANGUAGE

CODING – LANGUAGES

Use the key code below to decode the words. Each space is one letter. Challenge yourself to go as quickly as you can. All of these words are in the category: **LANGUAGES**.

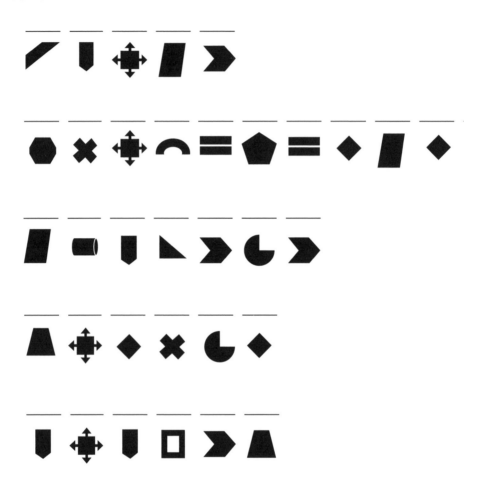

KEY CODE

A	B	C	D	E	F	G	H	I	J	K	L	M

N	O	P	Q	R	S	T	U	V	W	X	Y	Z

SYMBOL CODING 5

Write the number that corresponds to each symbol in the empty boxes below. Challenge yourself to do this as quickly as you can, while maintaining accuracy. Do not do all of one symbol at a time, complete each box in a row moving from left to right, and then continue to the next line.

KEY CODE

1	2	3	4	5	6	7	8	9
◺	⊤	\	⬭	◇	✚	↩▲	▭	✕

2	9	8	5	1	4	7	3	6	8
6	3	1	7	2	5	9	8	2	1
2	4	6	9	5	3	4	7	1	8
1	5	2	4	7	9	3	6	8	3
3	6	7	8	3	4	9	1	2	5
5	9	1	4	2	7	5	9	8	6
4	1	6	8	2	9	3	5	4	2
7	9	3	1	4	2	7	8	5	6

LOGIC WORD PROBLEMS 5

These word problems require you to use the process of elimination to find the answer. It helps to use the grid below.

X = No, not the correct answer; O = Yes, the correct answer

Using the clues, fill in the grid with X's and O's. When there is only one choice left in a row or column, put an O there. Because it is the only option left, it is the correct answer. If a clue tells you the correct choice, you can put an O in that box and put X's in the rest of the column and row because the other options cannot be correct too. Work through all of the clues this way.

1. Jerry was landscaping his backyard and trying to bring in a lot of different colors. He wanted a fruit tree, a rosebush, a scrub with flowers, and a succulent plant with a bloom. Can you determine what color each item was?

	RED	ORANGE	YELLOW	PINK
FRUIT TREE				
ROSEBUSH				
SCRUB				
SUCCULENT				

CLUES
a. Apples are Jerry's favorite fruit, so he definitely wanted those in his yard.
b. The succulent did not have a pink or yellow bloom.
c. Jerry could not find a scrub with pink blooms.

REASONING

2. Each of Bonnie's grandchildren play a different sport. Can you determine who plays which sport?

	BASEBALL	SOCCER	BASKETBALL	GOLF
BILLY				
KEVIN				
SANDRA				
KELLY				

CLUES

a. Kevin wants to be a pro baseball player when he grows up.

b. Sandra has never wanted to play any team sport.

c. Kelly can not use her hands in her sport.

MISMATCH 3

Pick out the one item that does not fit the category, and explain the *reason* why it does not fit.

1. Jazz, Opera, Classical, Guitar

    Mismatch item_____

    *Reason*_____

2. Sailboat, Ski boat, Kayak, Canoe

    Mismatch item_____

    *Reason*_____

3. Oboe, Flute, Piano, Clarinet

    Mismatch item_____

    *Reason*_____

4. Roses, Lilies, Daisies, Thistle

    Mismatch item_____

    *Reason*_____

5. Blue, Hues, Tints, Shades

    Mismatch item_____

    *Reason*_____

6. Echo, Movement, Hum, Buzz

    Mismatch item_____

    *Reason*_____

7. Volume, Sound, Clamor, Bright

    Mismatch item_____

    *Reason*_____

EXECUTIVE FUNCTIONING

8. Painter, Drawer, Sculptor, Illustrator

Mismatch item_____

*Reason*_____

9. Ornaments, Jewelry, Ribbon, Garland

Mismatch item_____

*Reason*_____

10. Loop, Ring, Clang, Jingle

Mismatch item_____

*Reason*_____

11. Seeds, Juice, Nectar, Sap

Mismatch item_____

*Reason*_____

12. Store, House, Apartment, Studio

Mismatch item_____

*Reason*_____

13. Mandate, Inquire, Query, Probe

Mismatch item_____

*Reason*_____

14. Lift, Boost, Raise, Advance

Mismatch item_____

*Reason*_____

15. Spaniel, Fox, Hound, Retriever

Mismatch item_____

*Reason*_____

16. Pretzels, Nuts, Peppers, Chips

Mismatch item_____

*Reason*_____

17. Headland, Island, Peninsula, Cape

Mismatch item_____

*Reason*_____

PARTS OF A WHAT? 3

Put these words into the most correct category.

lyrics   board   cards   a toast
cover   harmony   applause   rules
chapters   speech   players   characters
decorations   instruments   chorus   index

1. Parts of a book

   _____   _____

   _____   _____

2. Parts of a game

   _____   _____

   _____   _____

3. Parts of a ceremony

   _____   _____

   _____   _____

4. Parts of a song

   _____   _____

   _____   _____

REARRANGE THESE

Rearrange the letters of these words to create a new word.

1. Friend _____
2. March _____
3. Talks _____
4. Eager _____
5. Meats _____
6. Ought _____
7. Peaks _____
8. Brief _____
9. Field _____
10. Verse _____
11. Melon _____
12. Ports _____
13. Shelf _____
14. Grate _____
15. Hooks _____
16. Needs _____
17. Votes _____
18. Hoses _____
19. Items _____
20. Night _____
21. Relay _____
22. Roses _____
23. Shout _____
24. Lapse _____
25. Ocean _____
26. Warts _____
27. Siren _____
28. Panel _____
29. Spray _____
30. Parks _____
31. Races _____
32. Saint _____
33. Shrub _____
34. Study _____
35. Vases _____
36. Causes _____

TWO DEFINITIONS 5

Two definitions for the same word are given. Fill in the correct word that matches both definitions.

1. A large furry animal

   To carry a large load

   ANSWER _____

2. A walking stick

   An employee

   ANSWER _____

3. Power

   To state a possibility

   ANSWER _____

4. The edge of a river

   A place to store money

   ANSWER _____

5. To have permission to do something

   A month of the year

   ANSWER _____

6. A place to wash your hands

   To not float

   ANSWER _____

7. To stumble

   A vacation

   ANSWER _____

8. The noise of a clock

   A parasite

   ANSWER _____

9. The stem of a plant

   To follow

   ANSWER _____

"L" WORDS

Using two clues, fill in the correct word that begins with "L."

1. To strike with a whip

   Eyelid

   ANSWER _____

2. A fine knitted fabric

   A part of a sneaker

   ANSWER _____

3. To be in charge

   To take someone by the hand

   ANSWER _____

4. To go back in a chair

   A sloping position

   ANSWER _____

5. Behind schedule

   Near the end of a time period

   ANSWER _____

6. Most recent in time

   Final

   ANSWER _____

7. Attached to a stem

   To turn pages quickly

   ANSWER _____

8. It will be returned

   To contribute to

   ANSWER _____

9. Unable to find your way

   Can't be recovered

   ANSWER _____

10. To overlap sheets of a substance

    A covering

    ANSWER _____

11. A narrow horizontal strip of paper attached to an object to describe it

    A company that produces music

    ANSWER _____

12. To go away from

    To allow to remain

    ANSWER _____

LANGUAGE

13. A traditional story
A famous person

ANSWER _____

14. Legitimate

Permitted by law

ANSWER _____

15. Probably

Might happen or be true

ANSWER _____

16. Makes things visible

Ignite

ANSWER _____

MATCHING CLUES 8

Match two of the word-parts to make a word that fits the clue. Each word-part is used only once.

key   bas   oke   nk

ket   bla   don   br

1. _____ carries things

   _____ bare or plain

   _____ out of money

   _____ a hoofed mammal

eal   ely   ker   ke

hi   app   ep   lik

2. _____ climbs mountains

   _____ an urgent request

   _____ to retain possession

   _____ probable

LANGUAGE

ONE COMMON LETTER 2

Scan each line to find the one letter each word has in common. Challenge yourself to go as quickly as you can.

Example: baker and milk both have "k"

					COMMON LETTER
1. debtor	fabric	abroad	harbor	phobic	_____
2. bestow	growth	fellow	newest	reward	_____
3. eagle	forget	digest	jingle	malign	_____
4. belief	citrus	avidly	filter	hobbit	_____
5. funder	ground	extinct	inhale	lineage	_____
6. Frisbee	gators	hinder	inward	longer	_____
7. savor	cavity	evict	gravel	wolves	_____
8. lumbar	insult	jurors	mumble	outrun	_____
9. fajita	hijack	deject	adjoin	unjust	_____
10. filter	adopt	busted	country	invite	_____

PROCESSING SPEED

CREATE YOUR OWN FAMILY TREE

Fill in the names of your family in the appropriate positions. Add or take away more children or grandchildren as needed. If you have great-grandchildren, add them too.

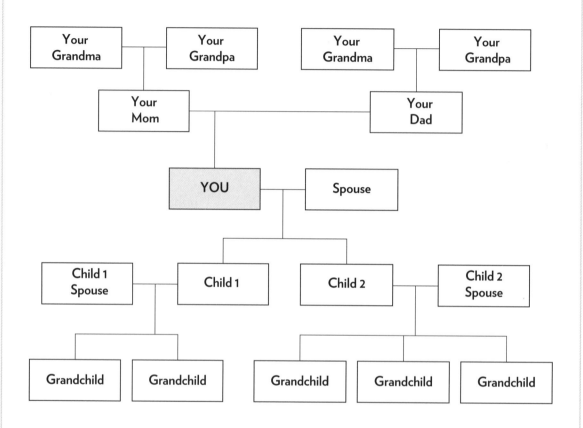

MEMORY

AN INVITATION– KEEP GOING!

SO HOW DO you feel after 201 exercises for your brain? Do you feel like you can think a little clearer, a little faster? Well then keep going! Your brain exercise regimen should not stop here. Research supports that brain stimulation must be regular and longterm in order for it to make a real difference. Just like physical exercise, we don't stop after a few months and expect the benefits to last. You must keep challenging your brain. Find unique and novel activities in which to engage. From simple tasks like driving a different way home to more difficult tasks like learning a new instrument, do all you can to stimulate your brain. We can often live on autopilot, just going through the motions of habit. Break your habits! Try new things! If you have never done crafts before, try painting or making pottery. Every small action counts towards building up brain strength!

You really can keep your brain stronger for longer!

ANSWERS

GRANDCHILDREN COMPARISONS pages 2–3

1. 1st Melanie, 2nd Patrick, 3rd Jimmy, 4th Cathy
2. 1st Lucy, 2nd Tom, 3rd Sally, 4th Amber
3. 1st Kate, 2nd Joe, 3rd Henry
4. 1st Marie, 2nd Neil, 3rd Yvonne, 4th Albert
5. 1st Robert, 2nd Olivia, 3rd Tamra, 4th Louie
6. 1st Vivian 44 pts, 2nd Eva 36 pts, 3rd William 32 pts

TWO DEFINITIONS 1 page 4

1. Box
2. Shade
3. Trunk
4. Bright
5. Foot
6. Rock
7. Punch
8. State

MATCHING CLUES 1 page 5

1. Banjo, rebel, jewel, joint
2. Joke, ajar, bake, back

SEQUENCING ITEMS 1 pages 6–7

The answers listed can go in either direction.

1. **Smallest to largest:** Flea, Ladybug, Bumblebee, Butterfly
2. **Shortest to longest duration:** Month, Semester, Fiscal year, Centennial
3. **Process of sculpting wood:** Chop, Carve, Sand, Paint
4. **Smallest to largest:** Millimeter, Centimeter, Meter, Kilometer
5. **Process of a buying house:** Credit check pre-approval, Offer, Escrow, Mortgage
6. **Process of starting a car:** Fasten seat belt, Check mirrors, Put into drive, Press gas pedal
7. **Process of baking:** Gather ingredients, Mix, Pour into pan, Bake
8. **Smallest to largest:** Pebble, Boulder, Hill, Mountain
9. **Process of digestion:** Mouth, Stomach, Small intestine, Large intestine
10. **Lifecycle of a butterfly:** Egg, Caterpillar, Cocoon, Butterfly
11. **Path of the sun:** Dawn, High noon, Dusk, Night
12. **Route of oxygen through the body:** Nose, Lungs, Blood, Body tissue
13. **Process of making yogurt:** Cow, Milk, Bacteria, Yogurt
14. **Process of getting accepted to college:** Application, Interview, Acceptance, Attendance
15. **Scientific method:** Hypothesis, Experiment, Analysis, Results

FAMILY TREE GAME 1 page 8

1. Leo
2. Susan
3. Mallory
4. Mallory and Mack
5. Mark
6. Loren

BOXED LETTERS – CARDS pages 9–11

1. Go Fish
2. Poker
3. Hearts
4. Gin Rummy
5. Spades
6. Crazy Eights

TWO-LETTER PLACEMENT 1   page 12

1. odor
2. adhere
3. brew
4. farm or form
5. dreary
6. average
7. case or care
8. hard or herd
9. cotton
10. plural
11. short
12. career
13. spray
14. orchard
15. secret
16. store
17. parent
18. argue
19. greed
20. early
21. coerce
22. marginal
23. origin
24. guard
25. insert
26. aversion
27. closet
28. scorn
29. laptop
30. thread
31. ceramic
32. toast
33. erase
34. cork

DECIPHER THE LETTER CODE 1   page 13

Message: When everything is coming your way, you are in the wrong lane.

WHAT'S THAT PHRASE? 1   pages 14–15

1. A dime a dozen
2. A piece of cake
3. An arm and a leg
4. It's all Greek to me
5. Back to the drawing board
6. Beat around the bush
7. Between a rock and a hard place
8. Break the ice
9. Burst your bubble
10. Close but no cigar
11. Cut to the chase
12. Down for the count
13. Down to the wire
14. Dropping like flies
15. Easy as pie
16. Elephant in the room

COUNT THE U'S   page 16

There are 72 U's.

AGING WORDS 1   page 17

1. Cage
2. Language
3. Collagen
4. Corkage
5. Blockage
6. Cottage
7. Garbage
8. Heritage

DOMINO ORDER 1   page 18

Here is one possible order:

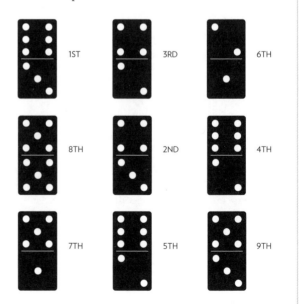

VENN DIAGRAM – LANGUAGES   page 19

1. 20 people
2. All three languages
3. 5 people
4. 70 people
5. 25 people
6. 65 people

DOT COPY 1   page 20

Go back and check yourself, or have a friend check your copied design.

SHAPE MATCH 1   page 21

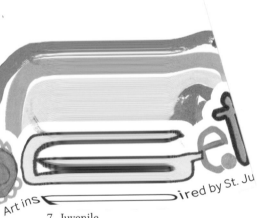

Art ins········ired by St. Ju···

7. Juvenile

Final message: Always remember you are unique, just like everybody else.

CODING – FAMILY   page 23

1. Cousin
2. Niece
3. Grandma
4. In-Law
5. Relative

MATCHING CLUES 2   page 24

1. Tarot, Degree, Siren, Rude
2. Rare, Step, Tarp, Late

FIRST AND LAST LETTERS 1   page 25

1. Crate
2. Restore
3. Press
4. Atone
5. Address
6. Peel
7. Untie
8. Note
9. Demo
10. Sheer
11. Oval
12. Trial

WORD MAZE – A LAZY SUNDAY   pages 26–27

1. Newspaper
2. Coffee
3. Donuts
4. Slippers
5. Long
6. Walk
7. Big
8. Meal
9. Family

START

A	P	T	R	W	Q	N	L	M	E	R	C
D	M	C	B	F	V	E	Y	K	P	D	O
G	N	O	L	S	E	W	S	P	A	H	F
W	H	K	J	R	H	X	T	H	L	E	F
A	L	K	Y	E	B	L	Y	O	D	E	Y
H	R	B	P	P	C	H	M	N	K	D	R
L	W	I	L	S	S	T	U	W	H	V
Q	Q	G	M	E	Q	L	K	A	C	B	Q
J	R	C	P	A	L	F	P	M	U	Y	P
O	L	N	B	V	F	A	C	B	S	O	T
M	A	S	D	B	A	M	U	P	V	B	N
B	K	P	B	I	M	B	C	K	N	F	B
G	J	C	Y	L	U	V	V	V	K	L	V

END

LOGIC WORD PROBLEMS 1 page 28

1. Billy – Dog
   Sally – Cat
   Cathy – Gerbil
   John – Fish
2. Irma – Banana
   Betty – Grapes
   Ralph – Orange
   Jim – Apple

MIDDLE LETTERS 1 page 29

1. Atom
2. Outer
3. Agree
4. Arena
5. Dart
6. Alone
7. Sweep
8. Aroma
9. Slept
10. Oxen
11. Value
12. Stare

BAGS OF WORDS page 30

1. Bagel
2. Airbag
3. Baguette
4. Handbag
5. Windbag
6. Beanbag
7. Cabbage
8. Saddlebag

ALLITERATION – PEOPLE page 31

There is no one correct answer. As long as every word starts with the same letter you got it right.

TRUE OR FALSE FACTS 1 pages 32–33

1. True
2. False
3. False
4. True
5. False
6. True
7. False
8. True
9. False
10. False
11. True
12. False
13. False
14. False
15. False
16. True
17. True
18. True
19. True
20. True
21. False
22. True
23. False
24. True

SYMBOL CODING 1 page 34

Go back and check yourself, or have a friend check your answers.

LETTERS-TO-WORD MATCH 1 page 35

Acquit, Blouse, Busier, Calmer, Damsel, Detach, Finest, Harden, Magnet, Parent

THREE-LETTER PLACEMENT 1 pages 36–37

1. radar
2. slogan
3. aerobic
4. frosting
5. saltine
6. apparent
7. fanatic
8. instinct
9. bicycle
10. darken
11. sales, dares, tines, or fanes
12. reverent
13. infant
14. accusal
15. matinee
16. boundary
17. elegant
18. salad
19. arrogant
20. retina
21. bicker, tinker, or darker
22. organize

23. salvage
24. tingle
25. profane
26. strength
27. darling
28. cubical
29. organ
30. fancy
31. outing
32. biceps
33. wrench
34. salute

ONLY THREE CLUES page 38

1. Basement
2. Park
3. Towel
4. Vacuum
5. Bottle

WHAT'S THE CATEGORY? 1 page 39

1. **Hardware store:** cabinet handles, ladder, wall mounts, concrete mix, floor wax, duct tape
2. **Park:** hikers, strollers, poison ivy, landmark, slide, fire pit
3. **Office:** printer, paper weight, books, calculator, to-do list, stamps

UNITS OF TIME 1 pages 40–41

1. 240 minutes
2. 9,000 seconds
3. 5 hours
4. 9:00 p.m.
5. 6:00 a.m.
6. 10:00 a.m.
7. 10:50 a.m.
8. 2 hours and 20 minutes, 10:10 a.m.
9. Since the flight time is 3 ½ hours you can't catch the 1:00 p.m., you'll have to take the 7:50 p.m. flight.
10. 1 hours and 47 minutes, 12:22 p.m.
11. 2 hours and 15 minutes, 4:15 p.m.
12. 8:00 – 10:00 p.m.

"B" WORDS pages 42–43

1. Buzz
2. Blow
3. Box
4. Buck
5. Buff
6. Back
7. Bow
8. Badger
9. Band
10. Bat
11. Bend
12. Blue
13. Board
14. Blush
15. Book
16. Brittle
17. Broke
18. Bait

WHAT IS THIS CALLED? page 44

1. Clothespin
2. Teddy bear
3. Pom-poms
4. Quilt
5. Bicycle
6. Fossil
7. Cricket or grasshopper
8. Fishing
9. Checkmate
10. Credit card
11. Cross-country skiing
12. Closed captioning

DOMINO ORDER 2 page 45

Here is one possible order:

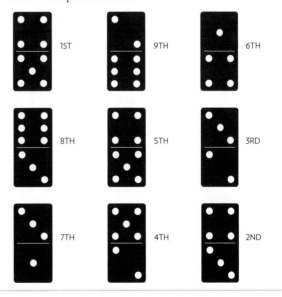

VENN DIAGRAM – BOOKS   page 46

1. 135 people
2. Romance
3. 0 people
4. 165 people
5. 75 people
6. 135 people

DECIPHER THE LETTER CODE 2   page 47

Message: Half of the people in the world are below average.

AGING WORDS 2   page 48

1. Mortgage
2. Salvage
3. Courage
4. Foliage
5. Marriage
6. Shortage
7. Manager
8. Sabotage

COUNT THE T'S AND P'S   page 49

There are 22 T's and 19 P's.

MISMATCH 1   pages 50–51

1. A tooth is not a type of store.
2. An eagle does not have four legs.
3. An apple is not a vegetable.
4. A shark lives in water, not on land.
5. A parrot is the only one that flies.
6. A coloring book is not a construction toy.
7. An eraser does not write.
8. Golf is not a team sport.
9. Dissolve is not a beginning.
10. Admission is not an object/way to get into house.
11. Separate is not a noun to name a thing.
12. Various does not mean one.
13. Inch is not a fluid measurement.
14. Vegetables do not have to be cooked first before eating.
15. A resort is not mandatory for skiing.
16. Helicopters are not in space

SIMILAR PROPERTIES   page 52

1. Have scales
2. Made of H_2O
3. Natural disasters
4. Can be cracked
5. Keep things together
6. Can be used to purchase items
7. Should be followed
8. Seasons
9. Must aim for them, or can hit them
10. Christmas decorations
11. Have caps
12. Grow on a stalk

BOXED LETTERS – GAMES   pages 53–55

1. Monopoly
2. Battleship
3. Scrabble
4. Chess
5. Charades
6. Pictionary

LETTER TRANSFER 2   pages 56–57

1. Orange
2. Declaration of Independence
3. Pennsylvania
4. New Orleans
5. Hershey's
6. Einstein
7. May

Final message: When it comes to thought, some people stop at nothing.

PROFESSIONAL CHARACTERISTICS   page 58

1. CEO: articulate, ability to delegate, confident
2. Artist: creativity, spontaneous, inspired
3. Physician: logical, empathetic, thorough
4. Soldier: courage, loyal, endurance
5. There are no right or wrong answers!

CALCULATION WORD PROBLEMS 1   page 59

1. 3 baking cups
2. 7 stickers each, 2 are left over
3. 19 pages for 20 days and 20 pages for 10 days
4. $250
5. 16 birds
6. 21 feet, 0 inches

CALENDAR QUIZ 1   pages 60–61

1. Wednesday the 9th
2. Sunday the 13th
3. Tuesday the 22nd
4. Tuesday the 22nd

A BIT OF WORDS   page 62

1. Orbit
2. Rabbit
3. Habit
4. Debit
5. Prohibit
6. Exhibit
7. Arbitrary
8. Inhabit

WHAT COMES NEXT?   page 63

1. Blue – ROYGBIV color spectrum order
2. Sol – Musical tone order
3. King – Hierarchy of royalty
4. Decade – Lengths of times
5. Continent – Locations, small to large
6. Scream – Voice volumes
7. Full house – Rank of poker hands
8. Shoulder – Joints, working up the arm
9. Queen – Rank order of chess pieces

PLACEMENT OF LETTERS 1   pages 64–65

1. ecology
   amplify
   infancy
   fashion
   benefit
   tactful
   diffuse
   officer
2. perform
   clarify
   testify
   factory
   unfolds
   golfing
   waffles
   justify
3. refusal
   enlarge
   careful
   footage
   enforce
   brought
   finance
   traffic
4. selfish
   defense
   wishful
   fantasy
   diagram
   certify
   garbage
   helpful

ABBREVIATIONS AND ACRONYMS   page 66

1. Captain
2. United Nations
3. Association
4. Established
5. Grand Old Party
6. Absence without leave
7. Incorporated
8. Bachelor of Arts
9. Century
10. Kilogram
11. Pound
12. District of Columbia
13. Carbon copy, cubic centimeter, chief clerk, closed-captioned, common carrier, community college, and country club
14. Limited
15. Miles per hour
16. Colonel
17. North Atlantic Treaty Organization
18. Ounce
19. Street or saint

LETTERS-TO-WORD MATCH 2   page 67

Active, Actual, Bounce, Bleach, Canopy, Cashew, Ethics, Factor, Mascot, Pickle

A BAN IN WORDS   page 68

1. Bandit
2. Cabana
3. Disband
4. Banquet
5. Abandon
6. Banister
7. Suburban
8. Banjo
9. Banal
10. Banish

SYMBOL CODING 2   page 69

Go back and check yourself, or have a friend check your answers.

UNITS OF TIME 2   page 70

1. 840 minutes
2. 18,900 seconds
3. 3 hours
4. 2:00 a.m.
5. 7:00 a.m.
6. 7:15 a.m.
7. 5:34 p.m., 26 minutes
8. 1:00 p.m. – 5:00 p.m. EST

DECIPHER THE LETTER CODE 3   page 71

Message: Middle age is when your age starts to show around your middle.

COUNT THE Y'S AND I'S   page 72

There are 32 Y's and I's

AGING WORDS 3   page 73

1. Eager
2. Voyage
3. Wreckage or carnage
4. Wage
5. Yardage
6. Engage
7. Message
8. Luggage or baggage

DOMINO ORDER 3   page 74

Here is one possible order:

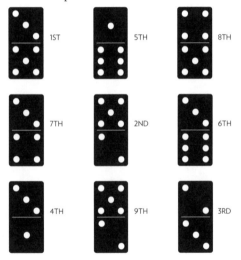

VENN DIAGRAM – MUSIC   page 75

1. 308 people
2. 66 people
3. 132 people
4. Rock
5. 132 people
6. 154 people

CALENDAR QUIZ 2   pages 76–77

1. Thursday the 8th
2. Tuesday the 27th
3. Thursday the 15th
4. Wednesday the 7th

DISCOVER THE PATTERN 1   page 78

1. 37, 60, 97, 157; each number is the sum of the 2 preceding numbers
2. 30, 38, 47, 57; add 3, add 4, add 5, add 6
3. 30, 18, 4; subtract 2, subtract 4, subtract 6, subtract 8
4. 88, 144, 234, 380; add the 2 preceding numbers plus 2
5. 3,584, 14,336, 57,344; multiply by 4 each step
6. 540, 1,080, 3,240, 6,480; multiply by 3, multiply by 2, multiply by 3, multiply by 2
7. 10, 6, 8, 4, 6; add 2, subtract 4, add 2, subtract 4
8. 26, 20, 13, 5; subtract 2, subtract 3, subtract 4, subtract 5
9. 34, 40, 46, 52, 58; add 6 each step
10. 205, 1,025, 1,030, 5,150; add 5, multiply by 5, add 5, multiply by 5

CLOCK QUIZ 1   page 79

1. 3:00 p.m.
2. 8:40 p.m.
3. 3:15 a.m.
4. 11:15 p.m.

TWO COMMON LETTERS 1   page 80

1. ji
2. pt
3. em
4. gh
5. pu
6. ew
7. lv
8. di
9. ka
10. rr

HOW MANY WORDS? 1   page 81

The answers in these lists are not exhaustive.

1. **Idiosyncratic**: idiot, dictionary, indicator, syndicator, rancid, crayon, dystonic, acidity, cystoid, scant, candy, acid, corn, crony, sync, city, coy, icy, cry, can, cod, in

2. **Scramble**: marble, calm, cable, blame, ramble, lamb, camel, clams, balm, carb, crab, scab, beam, lab, be, me

ALLITERATION – CELEBRITIES   page 82

There is no one correct answer. As long as every word starts with the same letter you got it right.

TWO DEFINITIONS 2   page 83

1. Rare
2. Polka
3. Range
4. Over
5. Row
6. Saw
7. Coast
8. Fly

A BID ON WORDS   page 84

1. Abide
2. Morbid
3. Forbid
4. Libido
5. Rabid
6. Counterbid

IMAGES MEMORY 1   pages 85–86

Shell, Towel, Umbrella, Starfish, Shovel, Flip-flops

WHAT IS THIS LOCATION?   page 87

1. Cape Canaveral
2. Mount Everest
3. Anaheim, California
4. Philadelphia, Pennsylvania
5. New Orleans
6. San Antonio, Texas
7. Yellowstone
8. Lake Superior
9. Chicago, Illinois
10. South Dakota
11. San Francisco Bay
12. Pearl Harbor
13. Nevada
14. New York Harbor
15. Grand Ole Opry

COMPLETE THE WORD SEARCH 1   pages 88–89

1. Egg
2. Irony
3. Essential
4. Tab
5. Reno
6. Candid
7. Swift
8. Ponytail
9. Vest
10. Net

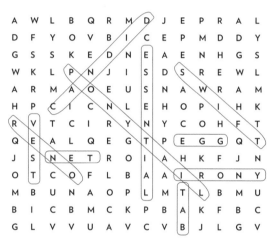

LETTER-NUMBER SUBSTITUTION CODE 1   page 90

1. Landmark
2. Camaraderie
3. Marionette
4. Outsmart
5. Marathon
6. Demarcate
7. Customary
8. Marginal
9. Grammar
10. Premarital

MISSPELLED WORDS 1   page 91

weigh, calendar, library, column, conscience, exceed, foreign, discipline, intelligence, address, noticeable, balance, until, weather, argument, believe

LOGIC WORD PROBLEMS 2   page 92

1. Helen – Chocolate
   Frank – Coconut
   Eddy – Custard
   Joyce – Raspberry
   Emma – Apple

2. Lou – Red bike
   Connie – Yellow car
   Stuart – Silver bus

WHAT'S THE CATEGORY? 2   page 93

1. **Sporting goods:** baseball, boots, fishing net, helmet, sweatshirts, umbrellas

2. **Mechanic:** taillight, grease, overalls, wrench, jack, seat cover

3. **Electronics:** headphones, camera, wire cable, power cord, book light, adapters

FIRST AND LAST LETTERS 2   page 94

1. Aisle
2. Rise
3. Gasp
4. More
5. Blade
6. Mascot
7. Test
8. Mane
9. Edit
10. Stir
11. Dear
12. Idea

ORDERED LETTERS 1   page 95

1. d
2. c
3. a
4. d
5. c
6. b
7. d
8. c

SHARED FOOD LETTERS   page 96

1. soup
2. beef
3. cake
4. salad
5. bread
6. raisin
7. cookie
8. cream
9. fish
10. pie

SHAPE ADDITION   page 97

1. c
2. b
3. d
4. b
5. c
6. a
7. c
8. d

PURCHASING PROBLEMS   pages 98–99

1. Remote control car and coloring book
2. Skillet, boiling pot, and serving dish
3. Cheese, deli meat, and crackers
4. Calculator and pencils
5. Beef, broccoli, and rice
6. Couch, armchair, and end table

DECIPHER THE LETTER CODE 4   page 100

Message: I always wanted to be somebody, but now I realize I should have been more specific.

COUNT THE VOWELS   page 101

There are 120 vowels.

AGING WORDS 4   page 102

1. Pageant
2. Rummage
3. Wager
4. Agenda
5. Image
6. Garage
7. Agent
8. Pages

DOMINO ORDER 4   page 103

Here is one possible order:

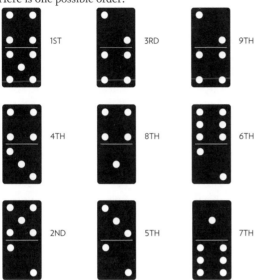

VENN DIAGRAM – TRANSPORTATION   page 104

1. 408 people
2. Train
3. 204 people
4. 170 people
5. 102 people
6. 102 people

NAME SOMETHING 1   page 105

The answers listed are not exhaustive.

1. P professions: physician, park ranger, psychologist, photographer, pharmacist
2. S professions: surgeon, scientist, social worker, surveyor, statistician
3. M books/movies: *Moby Dick*, *Macbeth*, *Madame Bovary*, *Malcolm X*, *Miracle on 34th Street*

LETTERS-TO-WORD MATCH 3   page 106

Absurd, Botany, Gravel, Hornet, Injure, Jockey, Kindle, Longer, Mobile, Pardon

WHAT'S NEXT? 1   page 107

1. c
2. b
3. a
4. b
5. a
6. c
7. b

CALCULATION WORD PROBLEMS 2   page 108

1. 34 total items; 18 flowers and 16 apples
2. 0 feet 5 inches
3. 5 pies
4. 4 gallons will last 16 days
5. 16 feet
6. 10 times

ACCOMPLISH THIS TASK 1   page 109

Here are two possible answers for each task

Keep papers together: staples, fold them together
Hang a picture: nail, tape
Join two pieces of wood: nails, glue
Grow a garden: outside in backyard, inside on kitchen window ledge
Build a tent: prepackaged tent kit for outdoors, indoors with bedsheets and pillows
Make a quilt: hand sew squares together, use sewing machine
Give a gift: hand it in person, mail it in box
Climb a hill: run up, walk up on knees
Travel across country: train, airplane
Pay for a purchase: cash, credit
Renew a library book: go into library in person, call and renew over phone

BAD WORDS   page 110

1. Badge
2. Forbade
3. Badminton
4. Badger
5. Badmouth
6. Troubadour

MATCH THE PARTS 1   page 111

1. dancer
   accuse
   leader
   formal
   botany
   parade
   canary
   reason
2. enlist
   cavity
   hoagie
   invent
   linear
   sodium
   active
   frolic

TWO COMMON LETTERS 2   page 112

1. fa
2. eb
3. ra
4. un
5. ct
6. pa
7. sc
8. ir
9. ey
10. rl

DISCOVER THE PATTERN 2   page 113

1. **14, 18, 22, 26**; add 4 each step
2. **80, 160, 320, 640**; multiply by 2 each step
3. **5, 7, 6, 8, 7**; add 2, subtract 1, add 2, subtract 1
4. **16, 14, 18, 16, 20**; add 4, subtract 2, add 4, subtract 2
5. **32, 128, 64, 256, 128**; multiply by 4, divide by 2, multiply by 4, divide by 2
6. **45, 42, 126, 123, 369**; multiply by 3, subtract 3, multiply by 3, subtract 3
7. **20, 20, 25, 25, 30**; add 5, multiply by 1, add 5, multiply by 1
8. **18, 23, 22, 28, 27**; add 2, subtract 1, add 3, subtract 1, add 4, subtract 1, add 5, subtract 1
9. **4, 20, 4, 24, 4, 28**; multiply by 2, divide by 2, multiply by 3, divide by 3, multiply by 4, divide by 4
10. **144, 720, 4,320, 30, 240**; multiply by 1, multiply by 2, multiply by 3, multiply by 4

COMPOUND WORDS 1   page 114

The answers listed are not exhaustive.

1. become, became, because, behold, beheld, begrudge, behead, belittle, befit, befriend, belabor, bemoan, beloved, beside, betaken, belong, begot, bebop, beset
2. inside, inward, into, inmate, inland, infield, income, indoors, infuse, inhale, insert, install, invest
3. outcome, outgrow, outside, outlaw, outrun, outfit, outback, outcast, outbid, outcry, outdone, outlook, outreach, outsource, outwit, outward

SYMBOL CODING 3   page 115

Go back and check yourself, or have a friend check your answers.

SEQUENCING ITEMS 2   pages 116–117

The answers listed can go in either direction.

1. **Writing process:** Outline, Rough draft, Editing, Final copy
2. **Water cycle:** Evaporation, Condensation, Precipitation, Accumulation
3. **Food chain:** Plankton, Fish, Bird, Cat
4. **Smallest to largest:** Paragraph, Flyer, Pamphlet, Novel
5. **Lowest to highest:** Foundation, Basement, Attic, Roof
6. **Chronological order:** Kennedy, Ford, Reagan, Bush
7. **Smallest to largest:** Rhode Island, Vermont, Ohio, Texas
8. **Electoral process:** Nomination, Voting, Ballot counting, Election
9. **Lowest to highest:** Ankle, Thigh, Waist, Forehead
10. **Order of buying:** Consumer, Store, Purchase, Take home
11. **Smallest to largest:** Blueberry, Mushroom, Avocado, Cantaloupe
12. **Chronological order:** Rosa Parks (1955), The Beatles (1964), *Apollo 11* (1969), Nixon resigns (1974)
13. **Judicial process:** Hearing, Trial, Sentencing, Appeal
14. **Smallest to largest:** Electron, Atom, Molecule, Element

WORDS THAT CAN   page 118

1. Vacant
2. Scandal
3. Canoe
4. Candid
5. Pecan
6. Candle
7. Cancel
8. Canvas

FAMILY TREE GAME 2   page 119

1. Ida
2. Nellie
3. His great-grandfather Gerald
4. Victor and Sam
5. Allie
6. Paul

MATCHING CLUES 3   page 120

1. Locket, mock, napkin, peak
2. Packet, task, prank, silken

WHAT'S THE CATEGORY? 3   page 121

1. **Closet:** zippers, hooks, hangers, photo albums, mothballs, hat box
2. **Science lab:** slides, eyewash kit, tubes, element chart, goggles, funnels
3. **Bank:** change, loans, interest, checks, vault, tellers

ORDERED LETTERS 2   page 122

1. C	4. C	7. B
2. B	5. A	8. B
3. D	6. D	

WHAT'S THE ITEM? 2   page 123

1. Dust
2. Clothespins
3. Straw
4. Button
5. Sponges

CLOCK QUIZ 2   page 124

1. 3:38 p.m

2. 6:30 a.m.

3. 9:20 p.m.

4. 5:30 a.m.

DECIPHER THE LETTER CODE 5   page 125

Message: A computer once beat me at chess, but it was no match for me at kickboxing.

COUNT THE CONSONANTS   page 126

There are 244 consonants.

WORDS FULL OF AWE   page 127

1. Declaw
2. Awestruck
3. Drawer
4. Flawed
5. Gnawed
6. Outlawed
7. Seaweed
8. Thawed

DOT COPY 2   page 128

Go back and check yourself, or have a friend check your copied design.

NAME SOMETHING 2   page 129

The answers listed are not exhaustive.

1. C countries: Canada, Chile, Costa Rica, Chad, Cambodia
2. G drinks: Gatorade, Gin, Ginger Ale, Grape juice, Grenadine
3. Y things: Yard, Yacht, Yarn, Yoke, Yo-Yo

LOGIC WORD PROBLEMS 3   pages 130–131

1. Sarah – second
   Walter – third
   Abby – fourth
   Neal – first
   Mallory – fifth
2. Lori danced the Lindy Hop with Leo.
   Amy danced the Jitterbug with Brian.
   Hank danced the Swing with Jane.
   Randy danced the Salsa with Natalie.

TWO DEFINITIONS 3   page 132

1. Leaves	5. File
2. Left	6. Ball
3. Nail	7. Pound
4. Fast	8. Mean

EDIT THE WORD 1   page 133

There could be several correct answers

1. Sable, Tale
2. Hunt, Hut
3. Lace, Ace
4. Sail, Ail
5. Fume, Use
6. Swan, Can
7. Barn, Bar
8. Bank, Tan

ACCOMPLISH THIS TASK 2   pages 134–135

Here are two possible answers for each task:

Dial a phone: phone number, something to say to the other person
Make coffee: coffeemaker, water
Grocery shop: shopping list, cart
Wrap a gift: money to buy the gift, someone to give it to
Go on a date: a plan, a location
Take a photo: camera, an interesting subject
Play a game: board game pieces, players

Feed your pet: pet food, bowl
Take a nap: bed, quiet
Play an instrument: talent, practice
Use a flashlight: batteries, dark
Write a check: money in the bank, signature
Wash your hair: shampoo, water
Keep a secret: a secret, strength of character
Ride a bike: a destination, inflated tires
Hem a dress: thread, needle
Go swimming: pool, swimsuit
Bake a cake: recipe, oven
Put out a fire: towel to cover over a small fire, baking soda to smother it
Replace a light bulb: light switch turned off, a new light bulb
Make ice: water, freezer
Walk around the block: sneakers, motivation
Tell a joke: a punch line, sense of humor

LETTER TRANSFER 3   pages 136–137

1. Federal
2. Navy
3. Heart
4. Texas
5. California
6. Hawaii
7. Swung

Final message: The road to success is always under construction.

A CUP OF WORDS   page 138

1. Occupation
2. Recuperate
3. Cupboard
4. Cupid
5. Hiccup
6. Occupy
7. Porcupine

CODING – OCCUPATIONS   page 139

1. Physician
2. Teacher
3. Accountant
4. Electrician
5. Pilot

LOGIC WORD PROBLEMS 4   pages 140–141

1. Sally – Jack of Hearts
   Rick – Ace of Spades
   Jay – King of Diamonds
   Beverly – Queen of Clubs

2. Harry – Lawn chair
   Emma – Scissors
   Joanne – Hammer
   Leo – Door hinge
   Diane – Wrench

ORDERED NUMBERS 1   page 142

1. c
2. a
3. d
4. b
5. d
6. d
7. a
8. c

MATCHING CLUES 4   page 143

1. Sketch
   Shiver
   Spark
   Think
2. Slick
   Yank
   Wicker
   Yoke

START HERE – END THERE   pages 144–145

There are many correct answers. For each answer just one example of an answer is given. You can check your answers with a calculator.

1. 2 + 18 – 5 = 15; 2 x 3 + 9 = 15; 2 / 2 + 14 = 15
2. 3 + 15 – 1 = 17; 3 x 3 + 8 = 17; 3 / 1 + 14 = 17
3. 4 + 20 – 2 = 22; 4 x 3 + 10 = 22; 4 / 2 x 11 = 22
4. 5 + 50 – 7 = 48; 5 x 8 + 8 = 48;
   5 x 30 / 3 - 2 = 48
5. 6 + 70 – 2 = 74; 6 x 6 x 2 + 2 = 74;
   6 x 25 / 2 - 1 = 74
6. 7 + 82 – 1 = 88; 7 x 11 + 11 = 88;
   7 x 20 / 2 + 18 = 88
7. 8 + 30 – 8 = 30; 8 x 5 – 10 = 30;
   8 x 10 / 2 - 10 = 30

8. 9 + 20 − 4 = 25; 9 x 3 − 2 = 25;
   9 x 4 / 2 + 7 = 25

9. 10+40-2=48; 10x4+8=48; 10/ 2x9+3 = 48

10. 12 x 6 − 10 = 62; 12 / 2 x 10 + 2 = 62;
    12 + 50 = 62

11. 15 x 6 − 4 = 86; 15 / 2 x 12 − 4 = 86;
    15 x 4 + 26 = 86

12. 24 x 3 + 20 = 92; 24 / 2 x 8 − 4 = 92;
    24 x 4 - 4 = 92

WORDS THAT FIT   page 146

1. Benefit
2. Misfit
3. Outfit
4. Profit
5. Retrofit
6. Graffiti
7. Befitting
8. Fitness

LETTERS-TO-WORD MATCH 4   page 147

Anchor, Attach, Cactus, Charge, Palace, Launch,
Orchid, Scenic, Secret, Tickle

SYMBOL CODING 4   page 148

Go back and check yourself, or have a friend check
your answers.

SUNNY WORDS   page 149

1. Sundae
2. Sunken
3. Sunbathe
4. Unsung
5. Sundress
6. Sunscreen or sunblock
7. Tsunami
8. Sundial

CALENDAR QUIZ 3   pages 150–151

1. Sunday the 14th
2. Saturday the 6th
3. Wednesday the 24th
4. Wednesday the 10th

TWO COMMON LETTERS 3   page 152

1. eg
2. lo
3. in
4. ru
5. ft
6. sr
7. ia
8. bl
9. tr
10. ic

CLOCK QUIZ 3   page 153

1. 9:45 p.m.

2. 4:00 a.m.

3. 7:05 a.m.

4. 12:50 p.m.

HOW MANY WORDS? 2   page 154

The answers in these lists are not exhaustive.

1. **Accoutrement:** accruement, accrue, counteract,
   recontact, contact, utterance, accent, contract,
   concrete, create, account, centrum, romance,
   concert, acumen, concur, cancer, accent, menace,
   occur, cameo, cream, came, coma, can, cue.

2. **Gardening:** danger, gander, anger, enrage,
   grading, ranging, grinned, edging, dagger, grand,
   gang, dang, aged, egg, gig, dig, in.

FURRY WORDS   page 155

1. Sulfur
2. Unfurl
3. Furnace
4. Furious
5. Refurbish
6. Furniture
7. Furlough

MIDDLE LETTERS 2 page 156

1. Smile
2. Hen
3. Echo
4. Utensil
5. Deli
6. Emotion
7. Aches
8. Seasons
9. Path
10. Saltine
11. Chat
12. Speed

MEMORY CROSSWORD 1 pages 157–158

Near, Amuse, Battle, Repair, Sender, Casino

IMAGES MEMORY 2 pages 159–160

Visor, Passport, Suitcase, Toothbrush, Compass, Wallet

DOT COPY 3 page 161

Go back and check yourself, or have a friend check your copied design.

"D" WORDS pages 162–163

1. Dot
2. Date
3. Detail
4. Dial
5. Direct
6. Dissolve
7. Domestic
8. Down
9. Draw
10. Drop
11. Drive
12. Dust
13. Decline
14. Depress
15. Dull
16. Dive
17. Dose
18. Deck

WORD MAZE – PATRIOTIC pages 164–165

1. Declaration
2. Freedom
3. Independence
4. Pledge
5. Allegiance
6. Justice
7. Duty
8. Veteran

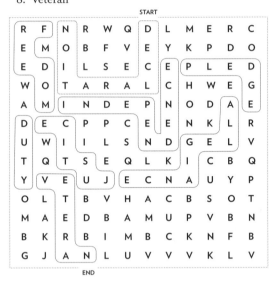

BETTING WORDS page 166

1. Better
2. Betray
3. Sorbet
4. Between
5. Betrothal
6. Alphabet
7. Diabetes

SHAPE MATCH 2 page 167

1. 4th and 7th shapes match
2. 2nd and 5th shapes match
3. 1st and 7th shapes match
4. 4th and 7th shapes match
5. 4th and 7th shapes match
6. 2nd and 4th shapes match
7. 1st and 5th shapes match
8. 5th and 7th shapes match

TRUE OR FALSE FACTS 2   pages 168–169

1. False	13. False
2. True	14. True
3. True	15. False
4. False	16. False
5. True	17. True
6. False	18. True
7. False	19. True
8. False	20. True
9. True	21. False
10. False	22. False
11. True	23. True
12. False	24. False

MISMATCH 2   pages 170–172

1. A Jet Ski is not for land transportation.
2. Mix is not a way to cut meat.
3. Ham is not a type of beef steak.
4. A fountain is not a form of water.
5. Waves are not a water mass.
6. A stream is not something you walk on.
7. A sheep is not a baby animal.
8. A report might not be based on facts/truth.
9. Reality is not made up or invented.
10. A manuscript is not a publicly distributed document.
11. An answer is not an emotional reaction or feeling.
12. Branch is not a family word.
13. Ocean is not an object you take to the beach.
14. Short-stop is not a football position.
15. Armor is not a weapon.
16. Seattle is not a state.
17. Microscope is not an adjective.

WORDS FULL OF FUN   page 173

1. Function
2. Fund
3. Fungus
4. Funnel
5. Refund
6. Funeral
7. Malfunction

WHAT'S THE CATEGORY? 4   page 174

1. **Ocean:** sand, shells, coral, tide, wreckage, divers
2. **Hospital:** bandages, needles, insurance, medications, sheets, elevator
3. **Restaurant:** menu, cashier, spices, booths, utensils, oil

WHAT'S NEXT? 2   page 175

1. a	4. b	7. c
2. c	5. c	
3. a	6. b	

CALCULATIONS   pages 176–177

1. Ages are 2, 4, 6, 8, 10, 12, 14, 16, 18, 20
2. 80 seats
3. $200 per month
4. 3 yards
5. 6 pieces each
6. 30 planks of wood
7. 4 hours
8. 5 large tables and 2 small tables
9. 1 coat

HOW MANY WORDS? 3   page 178

The answers in these lists are not exhaustive.

1. **Prestidigitation**: Rest, Digit, Dig, It, On, Tad, Opt, Date, Diet, Drag, Den, Drip, Gate, Oat, Pie, Pig, Pin, Pine, Pear, Pare, Rap, Reap, Rid, Ride, Rat, Rise, Risen, Sit, Sip, Sir, Stir, Stand, Snap, Side, Sedation, Sedan, Tie, Tip, Tan, Trip, Tide, Tired, Riptide, Edition
2. **Mellow**: Meow, Low, Elm, Mole, Well, Moe, Owe, Owl, Woe

WORDS FULL OF INK   page 179

1. Think
2. Link
3. Sink
4. Stink
5. Drink
6. Tinker
7. Shrink
8. Wrinkle

TWO-LETTER PLACEMENT 2   pages 180–181

1. canine	6. calm
2. actual	7. faint
3. disco	8. factor
4. allow	9. gossip
5. inland	10. floral

11. labor
12. crispy
13. inside
14. kindle
15. fossil
16. local
17. sign
18. issue
19. dialogue
20. blank
21. desire
22. legal
23. local
24. enact
25. cousin
26. saliva
27. scarf
28. raise
29. plaque
30. grain
31. linear
32. fiscal
33. react
34. wise

ORDERED NUMBERS 2   page 182

1. b
2. c
3. d
4. a
5. c
6. d
7. d
8. b

ORDERED SYMBOLS 1   page 183

1. c
2. d
3. b
4. c
5. a
6. b
7. d
8. d

THREE-LETTER PLACEMENT 2   pages 184–185

1. endear
2. tartar
3. spouse
4. walker
5. brand
6. clear
7. house
8. altar
9. honor
10. bearing
11. errand
12. callous
13. seeker
14. start
15. north or earth
16. orange
17. weary
18. furious
19. kernel
20. heart
21. snore
22. cued
23. grand
24. rescue
25. serious
26. earth or north
27. bakers
28. starch
29. barbecue
30. rocker
31. unlearn
32. lousy
33. cranky
34. stars

ASKING WORDS   page 186

1. Mask
2. Flask
3. Task
4. Askew
5. Basket
6. Gasket

MATCHING CLUES 5   page 187

1. Cable, absorb, abrupt, ballad
2. Badger, ballet, barely, double

SHARED NATURE LETTERS   page 188

1. tree
2. beach
3. wind
4. leaves
5. lake
6. flower
7. mountain
8. breeze
9. rain

WORDS FULL OF AIR 1   page 189

1. Éclair
2. Despair
3. Chairman
4. Airbrush
5. Prairie
6. Solitaire
7. Impair
8. Millionaire

CALCULATION WORD PROBLEMS 3   page 190

1. 10:30
2. Yes
3. 19 adults
4. 33 flowers
5. 16 sodas
6. 640 copies of the flyer

"G" WORDS   page 191

1. Goal
2. Glad
3. Game
4. Grace
5. Guest
6. Groom
7. Graph
8. Grill
9. Guard
10. Gross

MATCH THE PARTS 2 page 192

1. behave	2. theory
gotten	worker
locket	bundle
rumors	devour
flavor	funnel
motive	injure
parody	nuance
colors	humble

OUR WORDS page 193

1. Tourism
2. Glamour
3. Source
4. Journey
5. Court
6. Savor
7. Adjourn
8. Courier
9. Gourmet or gourmand

PLACEMENT OF LETTERS 2 pages 194–195

1. change	3. gallop
agency	belong
region	orange
tongue	crunch
finger	during
magnet	slogan
voyage	growth
golden	legend
2. dialogue	4. engine
higher	timing
signal	gentle
ignore	harbor
vigor	bright
assign	origin
wagons	racing
mingle	loving

SOLUTIONS TO A PROBLEM page 196

Here are two possible solutions for each problem:

Feeling stressed out: punch a pillow, call a friend

Car won't start: make sure you have gas, call a tow truck

Can't find keys: backtrack your steps, get your spare set of keys you keep in safe place

Have a headache: take aspirin, take a nap

Late bill payment: send check immediately, call company and apologize

Electricity goes out: go to breaker box and switch breakers, confirm you paid electric bill

Burn your hand: run under cold water, put clean loose bandage over it

A fly in the kitchen: open door and let it fly out, hit with flyswatter

Neighbor's dog won't stop barking: call neighbor and complain, put in earplugs and ignore it

Lost your wallet: call and cancel debit/credit cards, close bank account

Double-booked appointments: call one entity to reschedule and apologize, use calendar

Locked keys in car: get spare set of keys kept in safe place, jimmy the door open

Squeaky door hinge: oil hinge; take out hinge pin, clean it, and replace it

ORDERED SYMBOLS 2 page 197

1. c
2. b
3. d
4. a
5. c
6. d
7. d
8. b

WORDS THAT HAM IT UP 1 page 198

1. Chameleon
2. Graham
3. Hammer
4. Sham
5. Hamper
6. Shampoo
7. Chamber
8. Hammock

COMPOUND WORDS 2 page 199

The answers listed are not exhaustive.

1. bedside, bedtime, bedrock
2. newspaper, newsstand, newsclip
3. ladybug, ladylove, ladyfinger
4. pigsty, pigpen, pigtail

5. handcuff, handshake, handbag

6. lifeless, lifesaver, lifelong

7. sandbag, sandbox, sandpaper

8. fireworks, fireman, fireplace

9. eyelet, eyebrow, eyeball

10. thumbtack, thumbprint, thumbnail

11. rainfall, rainbow, raindrop

12. moonlight, moonshine, moonbeam

13. buttercup, butterfly, butterball

14. bookworm, bookshelf, bookcase

15. doorbell, doorstop, doormat

16. headlight, headache, headstrong

SEQUENCING ITEMS 3 pages 200–201

The answers listed can go in either direction.

1. **Order of math education:** Algebra, Geometry, Trigonometry, Calculus

2. **Chronological order:** *The Tramp,* 1914; Rosie the Riveter, 1942; *I Love Lucy,* 1951; Marilyn Monroe, 1954

3. **Chronological order:** Amelia Earhart, 1932; United Nations founded, 1945; Moon landing, 1969: Berlin Wall, torn down 1989

4. **Lightest to darkest color:** Yellow, Orange, Blue, Black

5. **Shortest to longest time commitment:** Dialing a phone number, Reading a brochure, Running a marathon, Writing a novel

6. **Process of mailing a letter:** Write letter, Address envelope, Stamp, Put in mailbox

7. **Process of starting a campfire:** Dig hole, Gather kindling, Stack firewood, Light match

8. **Process of getting dressed:** Pants, Belt, Socks, Shoes (It can be any order you prefer as long as pants come before belt and shoes, and socks comes before shoes).

9. **Process of planting:** Dig hole, Place seed, Cover with dirt, Water

10. **Process of building:** Planning, Designing, Buying supplies, Constructing

11. **Slowest to fastest:** Walking, Jogging, Running, Sprinting

12. **Process to marry:** Courting, Vows, Reception, Anniversary

13. **Across the United States East to West:** Boston, New York, Nashville, Los Angeles

14. **Order of holidays during a year:** Valentine's Day, Labor Day, Halloween, Thanksgiving

15. **Process of purchasing an item:** Choose, Pay, Change, Receipt

MISSPELLED WORDS 2 page 202

acceptable, liaison, exhilarate, receipt, grateful, license, jewelry, rhyme or rhythm, accommodate, guarantee, sergeant, threshold, humorous, ignorance, millennium

TWO COMMON LETTERS 4 page 203

1. gh
2. lm
3. sk
4. fr
5. ab
6. bu
7. is
8. cy
9. he
10. ju

BLANK CROSSWORD page 204

Have a friend check your answers.

MATCHING CLUES 6 page 205

1. Before
   Belong
   Edible
   Humble

2. Labor
   Marble
   Obtain
   Ribbon

WORDS WITH OUT page 206

1. Routine
2. Sprout
3. Shout
4. Route
5. Snout

6. Youth

7. Payout

8. Scout

9. Boutique

PARTS OF A WHAT? 1   page 207

1. **Camera:** lens, flash, shutter, aperture

2. **Phone:** speaker, keypad, cord, receiver

3. **Car:** window, ignition, wheel, hood

4. **Boat:** deck, rudder, masthead, tiller

WHAT'S THAT PHRASE? 2   pages 208–209

1. Every cloud has a silver lining

2. Fish out of water

3. Go for broke

4. Go out on a limb

5. Goody Two-Shoes

6. Happy as a clam

7. Hard pill to swallow

8. Head over heels

9. In a pickle

10. Jack-of-all-trades

11. Jump the gun

12. Keep on truckin'

13. Knock your socks off

14. A mountain out of a molehill

15. My cup of tea

16. On cloud nine

17. Rain on your parade

LETTER TRANSFER 4   pages 210–211

1. Ivory

2. Diamond

3. Aldrin

4. Arizona

5. Peanuts

6. Jamaica

7. Golf

Final message: Age is a question of mind over matter:
If you don't mind, age don't matter.

COMPLETE THE WORD SEARCH 2   pages 212–213

1. Elope

2. Hay

3. Donate

4. Entrance

5. Genes

6. Ignore

7. Tame

8. Cent

9. Ladle

10. Robes

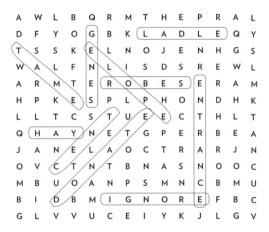

UPSIDE DOWN   page 214

1. C

2. B

3. D

4. C

HOT WORDS   page 215

1. Photo

2. Hotel

3. Shot

4. Hotline

5. Slingshot

6. Orthotics

7. Psychotic

8. Dichotomy

LETTER-NUMBER SUBSTITUTION CODE 2 pages 216-217

1. Applicable
2. Practice
3. Eradicate
4. Replicate
5. Despicable
6. Predictable
7. Education
8. Allocate
9. Revocable
10. Cabinet

TWO DEFINITIONS 4 page 218

1. Deck
2. Light
3. Rock
4. Staff
5. Grades
6. Note
7. Difference
8. Scale

FIRST AND LAST LETTERS 3 page 219

1. Tantrum
2. Solar
3. Atlas
4. Lead
5. Heard
6. Reign
7. Above
8. Satin
9. Line
10. Wish
11. Stain
12. Drop

CALENDAR QUIZ 4 pages 220–221

1. Sunday the 28th
2. Friday the 26th
3. Saturday the 13th
4. Tuesday the 30th

RAPPING WORDS page 222

1. Trap
2. Wrap
3. Strap
4. Rapid
5. Drape
6. Scrape
7. Entrap
8. Graphic

ONE COMMON LETTER 1 page 223

1. P
2. D
3. U
4. M
5. L
6. C
7. Y
8. K
9. H
10. F

MIDDLE LETTERS 3 page 224

1. Plea
2. Nice
3. Tent
4. Inner
5. Apple
6. Mimic
7. Negate
8. Lure
9. These
10. Crawl
11. Pedal
12. Toad

MEMORY CROSSWORD 2 pages 225–226

Marker, Accrue, Amoeba, Detail, Bushel, Sing

IMAGES MEMORY 3 pages 227–228

Swing, Pool, Fence, Lawn chair, Spatula, Barbecue grill

CALCULATION WORD PROBLEMS 4 page 229

1. A. $8.78
   B. $16.22 profit each
   C. $243.30 total profit
2. 96 strawberries
3. 257 people
4. 321 people
5. Yes

WORDS FULL OF AIR 2 page 230

1. Stairs
2. Hair
3. Fairy
4. Unfair
5. Dairy
6. Pair
7. Affair
8. Repair

MATCHING CLUES 7 page 231

1. Parade
   Patent
   Level
   Entree

2. Basket
   Erase
   Note
   Ideal

EDIT THE WORD 2 page 232

There could be several correct answers.

1. Rusty, Duty
2. Firm, Far
3. Fear, Ear
4. Shot, Hut
5. Fist, Fat
6. That, Hat
7. Hero, Her
8. Hair, Air

WHO IS THIS PERSON? page 233

1. Frank Sinatra
2. Dr. Spock
3. Winston Churchill
4. George Orwell
5. Rosa Parks
6. Alfred Hitchcock
7. John F. Kennedy
8. Andy Warhol
9. Johnny Carson
10. Martin Luther King Jr.
11. Thurgood Marshall
12. Neil Armstrong
13. Richard Nixon
14. Ted Turner
15. James Dean

TWO COMMON LETTERS 5 page 234

1. lo
2. mn
3. br
4. we
5. ld
6. hi
7. sk
8. rg
9. ot
10. ck

SHAPE MATCH 3 page 235

1. 1st and 4th shapes match
2. 2nd and 5th shapes match
3. 1st and 7th shapes match
4. 3rd and 7th shapes match
5. 2nd and 4th shapes match
6. 3rd and 5th shapes match
7. 2nd and 5th shapes match
8. 1st and 5th shapes match

WORD MAZE – NEWS pages 236–237

1. Headlines
2. Article
3. Front
4. Page
5. Column
6. Press
7. Reporter
8. Local

PARTS OF A WHAT? 2 page 238

1. House: pantry, staircase, attic, foyer
2. Classroom: rules, rulers, desks, notebooks,
3. Airplane: cockpit, passengers, wings, motor
4. Garden: path, fertilizer, fountain, sunshine

WORDS THAT HAM IT UP 2 page 239

1. Hamster
2. Shame
3. Champagne
4. Hamburger
5. Chamomile
6. Shambles
7. Champion
8. Hamstring

CODING – LANGUAGES   page 240

1. Farsi
2. Portuguese
3. Swahili
4. Creole
5. Arabic

SYMBOL CODING 5   page 241

Go back and check yourself or have a friend check your answers.

LOGIC WORD PROBLEMS 5   pages 242–243

1. Fruit tree – red
   Rose bush – pink
   Scrub – yellow
   Succulent – orange
2. Billy – basketball
   Kevin – baseball
   Sandra – golf
   Kelly – soccer

MISMATCH 3   pages 244–246

1. A guitar is not a type of music.
2. A ski boat has a motor.
3. A piano is not a wind instrument.
4. Thistle is not a flower.
5. Blue is not a description of color.
6. Movement is not a type of noise.
7. Bright is not something you hear.
8. A sculptor is not an artist who creates in two dimensions.
9. Jewelry is not hung on a holiday tree.
10. Loop is not a sound a bell makes.
11. Sap does not come from a fruit.
12. A store is not a place where you can live.
13. To mandate is not to ask a question.
14. To advance is not to move higher.
15. A fox is not a type of dog.
16. Peppers are not salty.
17. An island is not connected to land.

PARTS OF A WHAT? 3   page 247

1. Book: cover, chapters, characters, index
2. Game: board, cards, players, rules
3. Ceremony: decorations, speech, applause, a toast
4. Song: lyrics, harmony, instruments, chorus

REARRANGE THESE   page 248

1. Finder	19. Times
2. Charm	20. Thing
3. Stalk	21. Early
4. Agree	22. Sores
5. Teams or Steam	23. South
6. Tough	24. Leaps
7. Speak	25. Canoe
8. Fiber	26. Straw
9. Filed	27. Risen
10. Serve	28. Plane
11. Lemon	29. Prays
12. Sport	30. Spark
13. Flesh	31. Cares or Scare
14. Great	32. Stain
15. Shook	33. Brush
16. Dense	34. Dusty
17. Stove	35. Saves
18. Shoes	36. Sauces

TWO DEFINITIONS 5   page 249

1. Bear	6. Sink
2. Staff	7. Trip
3. Might	8. Tick
4. Bank	9. Stalk
5. May	

"L" WORDS   pages 250–251

1. Lash	9. Lost
2. Lace	10. Layer
3. Lead	11. Label
4. Lean	12. Leave
5. Late	13. Legend
6. Last	14. Legal
7. Leaf	15. Likely
8. Loan	16. Light

MATCHING CLUES 8   page 252

1. Basket
   Blank
   Broke
   Donkey

2. Hiker
   Appeal
   Keep
   Likely

ONE COMMON LETTER 2   page 253

1. b
2. w
3. g
4. i
5. s
6. r
7. v
8. u
9. j
10. t

CREATE YOUR OWN FAMILY TREE   page 254

Share your Family Tree with a friend or relative and have them review your work.

ABOUT THE AUTHOR

TONIA VOJTKOFSKY, PsyD, is a licensed clinical psychologist and sought-after specialist in cognitive disorders at the forefront of health care. Dr. Vojtkofsky received her masters and doctorate in clinical psychology from Rosemead School of Psychology, and did neuropsychological training at University of California, Irvine, Institute for Memory Impairments and Neurological Disorders as well as their Alzheimer's Disease Research Center. She is the founder of Cognitive Care Solutions in southern California, a clinic for people with MCI, mild dementia, as well as healthy older adults. In addition, Dr. Vojtkofsky has treated mood, psychotic, and cognitive disorders at Oregon State Hospital. She is a member of the American Psychological Association, USAgainstAlzheimer's, and a founding member of WomenAgainstAlzheimer's.

For more information visit CognitiveCareSolutions.com.